THE ATHLETE'S SIMPLE GUIDE TO A PLANT-BASED LIFESTYLE

The Athlete's Simple Guide to a Plant-Based Lifestyle

How to easily improve your health, performance, and longevity.
Works for non-athletes, too!

SUZANNA MCGEE

The Athlete's Simple Guide to a Plant-Based Lifestyle

How to easily improve your health, performance, and longevity.
Works for non-athletes, too!

First Edition Copyright © 2014 by Suzanna McGee
Photos Copyright © 2014 by Suzanna McGee
Copyediting by Janet Kolbu and Doree Gerold
Proofreading by Wendy Brynford-Jones
Cover art by Maria Rosetti
Zuzi Publishing

Library of Congress Control Number: 2013957735
First Edition, 2014
ISBN-10: 0-9829499-0-1
ISBN-13: 978-0-9829499-0-0
Published in the United States of America

Note: The health procedures in this book are based on the training, personal experiences, and research of the author. The information in this book is true and complete to the best of our knowledge. This book is intended only as an informative guide for those wishing to know more about health issues. Because each person and situation is unique, the author and publisher urge the reader to check with a qualified health professional before using any procedure where there is any question as to its appropriateness. In no way is this book intended to replace, countermand, or conflict with the advice given by your own physician. The ultimate decision concerning care should be made between you and your doctor. We strongly recommend following your doctor's advice.

Because there is always some risk involved, the author and publisher disclaim all liability in connection with the use of this book. Please, do not use this book if you are unwilling to assume the risk. Feel free to consult a physician or other qualified health professional. Seeking a second or third opinion is a sign of wisdom, not weakness.

Learn more information at: www.TennisFitnessLove.com

[D]

DEDICATION

To all the remarkable people out there who have decided to live long and healthy lives full of positive energy and who have the courage to do something different than our current society dictates.

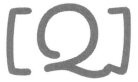

QUOTES OF PLANT-BASED ATHLETES

Carl Lewis
World Champion Sprinter with 9 gold and 1 silver Olympic medals

"I've found that a person does not need protein from meat to be a successful athlete. In fact, my best year of track competition was the first year I ate a vegan diet. Moreover, by continuing to eat a vegan diet, my weight is under control, I like the way I look. (I know that sounds vain, but all of us want to like the way we look.) I enjoy eating more, and I feel great."

***

Brendan Brazier
Former professional Ironman triathlete, author, and creator of the Vega line of food products and supplements

"Plant-based nutrition totally works for strength athletes, too, for building muscle. This is because plant-based food is alkaline-forming, and when you eat alkaline foods, it reduces inflammation, and if you reduce inflammation, you increase functionality. And more functional muscles have the ability to lift heavier weight. Lifting heavier weight is what builds bigger, stronger muscles. So, being vegan doesn't make you a stronger, better athlete, but it allows you to make yourself a stronger, better athlete. It allows you to work harder, and that's what ultimately makes you a better athlete. It's just facilitating your body's ability to work harder, more efficiently."

***

David Cartner

NFL player, Oakland Raiders

"As a professional athlete what I put in my body for breakfast, lunch, and dinner, are some of the most important decisions I make every day. I must ensure I'm consuming sufficient calories to keep full and have the energy to perform at my peak while not overloading and slowing my body down. My career depends on it. So many people are shocked when they learn that I fuel my body with a plant-based—vegan—diet. I'm just shocked that it took me 26 years to gain the wisdom to do it!"

***

Alexey Voyevoda

Russian bobsledder and world champion arm-wrestler, 2014 Olympic Gold medalist

"A plant-based diet keeps me light, flexible, and healthy. My body has become lighter, so to say 'clearer.' In my profession, flexibility and elasticity are incredibly important, and I increased both of these. And… now I almost never suffer from a cold or flu."

***

Robert Cheeke

Vegan Bodybuilder, Activist, Motivational Speaker, Author

"I definitely have more energy, an easier digestion, increased metabolism, and much reduced recovery time after workouts. I have less inflammation, can train harder and faster, and my heart and joints are much healthier—there is really nothing negative I can think of as being a vegan athlete."

***

Mac Danzig

Professional UFC Fighter

"I switched to an entirely vegan diet in 2004 for personal ethical reasons and was immediately surprised at how great I felt when training and competing. I recover faster from workouts and have more energy than I did before. For me, it is a simple, life-long decision. Not only do I feel physically better than ever, but I also have the satisfaction of knowing that I am not directly contributing to the industries that are so detrimental to animals, the environment and the people involved."

***

Venus Williams

Professional tennis player, a former World No. 1, 7 singles Grand Slam titles

"I had to change my diet. I had to do many changes. I've become a raw vegan, and I am not perfect, so I forgive myself when I make mistakes. I do a lot of juicing as well, a lot of wheat grass shots, lots of fresh juices and things like that. I have made huge improvements with raw vegan diet."

***

Timothy Bradley

WBO welterweight champion

"A vegan diet helps keep my body clean and it provides me with a tremendous amount of energy due to my body spending less energy breaking down foods like meats. This is a big key factor in my fitness. I told a reporter recently that I feel totally superior over any athlete who gets into the ring with me. The energy is always there. I feel so alive. My senses and reflexes are so acute. It's an incredible feeling. Rest, preparation, rest, hard work—but rest is very important. It gives you the right kind of balance. With a vegan diet you always have energy, so much that sometimes I have trouble sleeping at night. You feel light. You don't feel bulky or heavy. This would benefit any athlete in any sport."

***

Scott Jurek

Ultramarathoner, one of the most dominant ultramarathon runners in the world

"It's not like you wake up the next morning and feel ten times better. The changes are more gradual and you can see them better once you continue down the path for a while and then look back. In regards to competing and training I noticed my recovery times had shortened, that I was less injury prone, and had a higher level of energy. Above all, the major changes were in my relationship to food preparation and intake. I became very concerned not just about veganism, but about proper nutrition. I've come across many vegans who are still drinking soda pop. The point is you can be vegan and still have an unhealthy diet."

***

Patrik Baboumian
One of the planet's strongest men, Armenian-German strongman competitor, psychologist, and former bodybuilder

"Strength must build up, not destroy. It should outdo itself, not others who are weaker. Used without responsibility, it causes nothing but harm and death. I can lift the heaviest weights, but I can not take the responsibility off my shoulders. Because the way we use our strength defines our fate. What traces will I leave on my path into the future? Do we really have to kill in order to live? My true strength lies in not seeing weakness as weakness. My strength needs no victims. My strength is my compassion."

***

Rich Roll
Author, Ultra-Endurance Athlete

"I feel quite strongly that a nutrition program built entirely around plant-based foods and completely devoid of animal products is optimal. Conventional wisdom would say that an athlete cannot perform on plants alone, but I am living proof that this is false and I have ample research to support this position. Personally, I cannot overemphasize the difference this has made in my own life; a secret weapon for enhanced athletic performance and overall long-term wellness. In the last two years, I have not gotten sick or even suffered a cold. I have found that I am able to repair my body and recover well from workouts and am able to bounce back fresh day in and day out. Believe me, if I felt like I really needed to eat meat or dairy over the last 3 years, I would have. I just never felt like I really needed to."

***

James Lightning Wilks
Professional Mixed Martial Artist/Retired UFC Fighter, Winner of The Ultimate Fighter: United States vs. United Kingdom

"I spent over 1,000 hours looking at peer reviewed medical science and realized that a plant-based diet is superior and optimal for health and athletic performance."

***

Christine Vardaros
Professional Cyclo-cross Cyclist

"I am a professional athlete so I may prove by example that top sport can be successfully accomplished on a completely plant-based diet.... It is especially important to me that everyone knows eating vegan is simple and easy and requires only basic foods that can be found in any supermarket around the world. Go Vegan and No Body Gets Hurt!"

***

Greg Chappell
Cricketer, Former Australia Captain

"I think the turning point for me was an article that I wrote from the information from the research done at UCLA in California on their track and field athletes, about dairy products, and their fitness and general health on and off dairy products. And the upshot of the article was that these athletes perform better, they recovered better, they trained better, and they were 100% aerobically more fit off dairy products than on dairy products, and I thought Well, for half the training I can be as fit as I am now."

***

John Salley
Retired NBA Player

"I explain to athletes, you're supposed to be a well-oiled machine. You're supposed to be in better shape than the people watching you. You're supposed to be an unbelievable specimen of a human being. You have to treat your body different while you're performing. Think about how Serena Williams winded up having a heart situation, two years ago? Right? Her sister Venus had Sjögren's syndrome, They hired my friend Lauren Vanderpool to be their chef, because Lauren was one of the greatest chefs I ever met. Knows so much, really good at preparing food, raw-slash-vegan. And Serena's number one again. And Venus is playing with power again. And it has to be the food, what these two smart sisters decided they were going fuel their body with."

***

Pat Neshek
Major League Baseball Relief Pitcher

"After the 2007 season I had read so much I decided to become a vegan and get rid of all the animal products—meat and dairy... It really changed my career, and I thought, 'This might be something that helps me take my career to the next level.' And it wasn't the main reason, but I like knowing everything I eat was served in a humane way."

Robbie Hazeley
Veteran Bodybuilder

"Going vegan was instrumental in improving my all round health, stamina, freedom from injuries and ability to train more intensely. It was the turning point for me in so many ways."

***

Daniel Bryan
Pro Wrestler (WWE)

"So, anyway I started going vegan then, and this whole year my energy levels have been great, I haven't gotten any skin infections. Right now I'm 198 lbs which is the heaviest I've weighed since 2003… I'm stronger right now than I've ever been. I'm dead-lifting more than I ever have before."

***

…AND SOME NON-ATHLETES, TOO!

Bill Clinton
Former U.S. president

"I just decided that I was the high-risk person, and I didn't want to fool with this anymore. And I wanted to live to be a grandfather, so I decided to pick the diet that I thought would maximize my chances of long-term survival. The main thing that was hard for me actually—much harder than giving up meat, turkey, chicken and fish—was giving up yogurt and hard cheese. I love that stuff, but it really made a big difference when I did it. If you don't have the willpower to do it for yourself, do it for your loved ones. You have a responsibility to try to be as healthy as possible."

***

[C]

CONTENTS

SECTION 1: INTRODUCTION

SECTION 2: BASIC NUTRIENTS AND FOODS YOU CAN EAT

SECTION 3: EFFECTS OF NUTRITION ON THE BODY

SECTION 4: FOOD PREPARATION

SECTION 5: IMPORTANT NON-FOOD TOPICS

MEDITATION

APPENDIX: NON-RECIPES AKA RECIPE BLUEPRINTS

*

SECTION 1

INTRODUCTION

[2]   Suzanna McGee

[1]

WHY THIS BOOK?

"Good health is about being able to fully enjoy the time we do have. It is about being as functional as possible throughout our entire lives and avoiding crippling, painful, and lengthy battles with disease. The enjoyment of life is greatly compromised if we cannot see, if we cannot think, if our kidneys do not work, and if our bones are fragile or broken"

Dr. T. Colin Campbell, *The China Study*

For an athlete, good health is the most important prerequisite to maximum performance. Without a healthy body, you will never achieve your athletic potential.

We all like to eat and feel good, but we also want to be fit and healthy, and athletes want to perform at their best and win. Nutrition, more than ever, plays an important role in our well-being and in athletic performance. People and athletes search for different styles of eating to improve health and performance. Some styles may deliver quick results, but they don't last long. One simple and effective way that also makes you feel great is eating plants.

Whole foods plant-based nutrition is not a diet, but rather a lifestyle, a pleasurable way of living life, filling you with boundless energy and a sense of well-being. If you have any physical challenges or illness, you will notice that your body will start healing and recovering. If you need to lose some weight, you will drop the pounds almost in front of your eyes. If you already feel healthy, you will find more energy, restful sleep, and increased performance in your sport or in your life.

The purpose of this book is to give you the information that you need to adopt this lifestyle and to gain the above-described and many other benefits. This book is a simple guide, which is easy to understand for everyone at any level of nutritional knowledge, without complicated scientific studies or material. For readers who wish to delve deeper into the science of healthy eating, the appendix contains references to the works of some of the plant-based and lifestyle professionals that I admire.

After studying and consulting many plant-based experts and high performance athletes, I deeply believe that whole foods plant-based nutrition is the way to optimal health, longevity, and performance. If you have been flirting with the idea of becoming plant-based for any reason, such as health, performance, anti-aging, the cool factor, or just because a friend or spouse does it and they feel great, this book is for you. It will help you transition into the world of plants smoothly when you decide to do it.

I like to read the studies, research, and books from doctors and other successful people who appear to practice what they preach. Experts, who are fit, lean, radiant, and healthy motivate me and awaken my curiosity. I want to hear what they have to say, because they are doing something right. On the other hand, a bloated, overweight, and unhealthy-looking person, who preaches about diet for achieving longevity and health doesn't generate much respect in my eyes. As educated as he well may be, if he cannot help himself with his theories, how can he help anyone else?

Unfortunately, there are not very many medical doctors that believe in the power of healing with food, but fortunately, the numbers are steadily increasing. Nutrition is not taught in medical schools, but a lot of inquiring medical minds search for something better than medications to help their patients, because they often see that drugs don't work well in the long term.

There are hundreds of studies supporting or opposing any of the eating styles, and people are confused by all the contradicting information the media delivers: oil is good; oil is bad; carbs are great; carbs are bad; gluten or no gluten? The Paleo people argue that we were made, as gatherers and hunters, to eat meat, but the anthropologists find this is not correct because grains were part of our diets even back then. In this book, I will not decide who is right or wrong. I will not preach how plant-based nutrition is the best, because different people need and want different things in life. I only know that this lifestyle is right for me, for many of my students, and for many other athletes and non-athletes.

Considering how our modern western lifestyle has too many stressors and toxins in our lives and environment, plant-based nutrition is healing to the body, allowing the immune system to regain its strength and fight for its health on all cylinders. A healthy body performs optimally in all athletic endeavors. Nutrition is more important than one dares to believe. If you have decided to choose health, longevity, and improved performance, this book will help you on your journey toward a plant-based eating plan.

In this book, you will find a review of my many years' experiences and findings, which I have learned from the most prominent doctors, health professionals, athletes, nutritionists, and other spectacular and knowledgeable people who understand that food will heal and empower you.

You will learn what to expect during the transition and how to ensure that you are getting all the nutrients, vitamins, and minerals that you need for optimal health and performance. You will learn a number of different ways to prepare whole foods, and a few extremely simple and fast recipes, which I call non-recipes, because there are no exact items and numbers to follow, rather, just a blueprint for many simple combinations of tasty meals. You will find advice on keeping costs low and once you discover how extremely simple this plant-based lifestyle is, you will never want to go back.

[2]

WHY ME?

I have been an athlete since I was 9 years old. On my athletic journey of many different sports, I have experimented with countless nutritional trends and tendencies: sometimes just following the craze, but more often deliberately and empirically testing the theory. The scientist in me has been there since my youth, hand in hand with the athletic side.

I lived in the less-developed Czechoslovakia for 20 years. We were poor and ate "poor" food, such as beans, rice, oats, and breads. In the 1980s, I moved to Sweden where the industrialized food revolution had just started: highly processed foods, wrapped in beautiful colorful plastics and boxes. Coming from a poor country to this, I felt like I was in heaven. How exciting it was to buy powdered potatoes or pre-made cookies and just blend it with water, cook for 5 minutes in the microwave oven and here we go… the meal is ready to eat.

BODYBUILDING

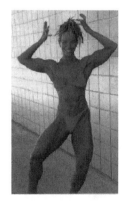

In the 1990s, I became a fitness competitor who transitioned into drug-free bodybuilding, winning the glorious title "Ms. Natural Olympia" champion. Because I was not using any illegal enhancement supplements, I had to be extremely disciplined, close to perfect with my nutrition so my body would recover from the intense training and dieting. For a female, reaching single-digit body fat levels translates to an intense and disciplined journey. My eating was healthy according to the popular standards of the late 90s.

All of my six to seven small daily meals contained chicken, fish, meat, or whey protein supplement. My protein intake in grams was very high, usually 1.5–2 times my body weight. During the three to four months' dieting period, in order to lean out for the competition, I experimented with all kinds of nutritional methods. I started with balanced nutrition, The Zone, which was very popular then, containing 30% of calories from protein, 30% from fat, and 40% from carbohydrates.

I experimented with ketogenic diets, where absolutely no carbohydrates other than 30 grams per day were allowed. Everything I ate was protein or fat. The few allowed grams of carbohydrates came from cheese, nuts, spreads, etc. A gram here, a gram there, it added quickly to 30 grams. This was a thought-provoking eating style, but it worked very well on those tough areas for women to lose fat: the lower buttocks and upper thighs. On the ketogenic diet, the fat melted beautifully.

My ketogenic eating was even more restrictive than the Atkins diet, which soon became relatively popular for the public. Atkins allows eating "crap." Not to sound offensive but by "crap" I mean processed meats, processed cheese, bacon, and fat-rich snacks. They all were ok to eat as long as they didn't contain any carbohydrates. A new era of foods emerged in the markets: the low-carb craze of all processed concoctions full of additives and chemicals, beautifully packed in inviting boxes and cans. Sometimes you couldn't even read the label because it looked like gibberish in a foreign language.

Nevertheless, people were happy: they were losing weight rapidly. Whenever you restrict carbohydrates, you lose a lot of weight initially, because every gram of carbohydrates (glucose) in your body binds 3 grams of water. If you lose one pound of carbohydrates, with them also goes their friend, three pounds of water. Even though you get dehydrated and don't perform well physically or mentally, you still feel excited by this rapid weight loss. Who cares about health in this situation? We like quick results and instant gratification don't we?

In the early 2000s, I achieved everything I wanted in my bodybuilding journey. I was capable of achieving 8% of body fat while being completely drug-free. I won numerous titles in addition to the prestigious "Ms. Natural Olympia". I competed in Greece, in the famous Olympic Stadium. My life was flowing, and I had everything under control.

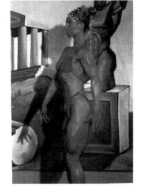

Nutrition was always a significant part of my personal research and I have always logged my food intake so I can learn and draw conclusions on what is working, how and when. In those days there were no smart phone apps or computer programs to make the task easy for you. My two masters degrees in computer science were put to great use: I created beautiful spreadsheets where I was logging and calculating everything I put in my mouth. Every evening, I preplanned all food for the next day, entered everything in my spreadsheet, looked up the nutritional values in the books, and calculated all the nutritional percentages. Once I achieved the numbers that I was satisfied with, my meal plan for the next day was ready. This was quite time consuming.

The next day, I cooked accordingly. Every food went through my little kitchen scale before it hit the pot. I ate 6–7 meals a day. According to today's plate size standards, my meals were very small, about 400–500 calories and I could easily call them "snacks" because they had the same number of calories as a large cola or donut.

I was extremely disciplined as I only ate what I planned. However, I also planned one cheat day every week and on that day I was like a human vacuum cleaner. There was no plan on what to eat. The only plan was to go to the grocery store on the morning of my cheat day, buy anything that my mind and body wanted (and during such strict eating, the mind wanted more than the body could handle) and I shopped and shopped: ice cream, nuts, cookies, these were my favorites. I was known to eat a half-gallon of Peanut Butter Fantasy ice cream topped with a pound of cashews.

On some of these cheat days I ingested 10,000 calories. This is nothing to brag about. It's crazy now when I think about how my body and mind over-indulged. The metabolism, suppressed by eating restricted calories, will get on fire again. After such a cheat day, you can only look forward to eating lightly and cleanly. This was a stage in my journey, and I do not recommend it. It was hard and too extreme. Nowadays, I believe in health more than anything.

TENNIS

In the early 2000s, I had a customer who was a tennis player. She always tried to seduce me into playing with her, and one day I succumbed. I felt quite challenged to hit the ball with the strings and into the court, not even thinking about hitting to a particular location. My client knew me very well and knew how passionately obsessive I get about everything. She was right: tennis got me hooked. I hated the feeling of not being able to control that little fluffy bouncy yellow ball and the hate-love tennis journey began.

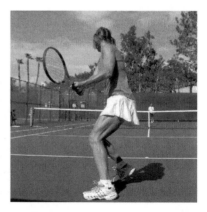

Soon I recognized that bodybuilding and tennis don't mix well. Training several times a day and eating every 2–3 hours was too complicated to organize when I was on the tennis court for a couple of hours and also needed time to digest the food. I was spending more and more time hitting the yellow ball, and less and less time cooking my six meals a day. My transition just happened. I felt that I had accomplished enough to my satisfaction in the bodybuilding arena. World beware: Ms. Natural Olympia is becoming a tennis player!

My training changed, my nutrition changed, and my focus changed. Obsessively passionate as I am, I was playing very regularly and if not with people, then practicing solo against the wall. Spending time with the fuzzy balls adjusted my eating habits and my routines. I began to eat less often, bigger meals and more carbohydrates. Carbohydrates are fuel for performance, easy to digest and easy for the body to access. I cannot even imagine stuffing myself with chicken breasts and broccoli before a tennis practice or match. I slowly drifted away from the bodybuilding; I loved tennis so much that I didn't care much about it anymore. I was still training in the gym, but even my training routines were slowly adjusting and changing.

Instead of splitting the muscle groups to be trained on different days, I began to do intense full body workouts that I repeated every other day, with many exercises to get the variation. I was 180 pounds when I started to play tennis. Within a couple of years, my body weight dropped and adjusted to lean and strong 160 pounds on my 6' tall frame, and has stayed there ever since. I was not the "muscle queen" anymore and many of my fans were disappointed, but I loved every step of my new journey.

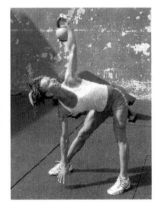

I thought I had all the training under control. After all of the years of training myself to achieve my titles, training others to realize their dreams, and continuously educating myself, I was on training autopilot. To my surprise, a few years into my tennis journey, I began to feel a little ache here, a little pinch there. One of those little aches in my left knee became more irritating than I would wish, and eventually became intolerable. This day was the turning point in my personal fitness and in my career as a trainer. I had discovered imbalances!

Some people discover God or other amazing things at various stages of their life journey, and their lives turn in a completely different direction. I had found imbalances, and they were the turning point for me. I adjusted my entire training program, educated myself even more, and was now training like a tennis player. I haven't had any injuries ever since. As my knowledge of new theories and science grew, my beliefs on the best diet changed significantly from looks-centric to health, longevity, and performance focused. A fit, light, and healthy body performs so much better and makes the mind feel great. In synergy, they add tremendous values to one's general well-being.

LIFE

My daily schedule is well planned and disciplined. Only in that way can I fit in all of the things I want and need to do. Learning and playing competitive tennis, training to be fit for tennis, stretching and doing injury preventive measures takes a lot of time and effort in addition to helping my clients to be fit and healthy and feel as great as I do. As I have done all my life, I always test new ideas and theories on myself. I test them thoroughly, writing down all the results, analyzing them and either discarding or keeping, while adjusting them with all the other theories. Ultimately, I have the best concoction of practices and systems that maximally improve both performance and health. I always continue to adjust them as new knowledge is attained.

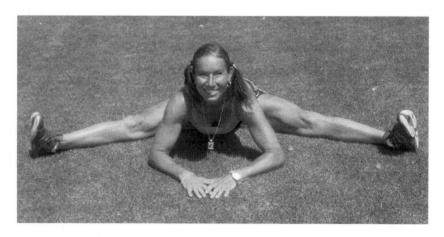

Nevertheless, there is one unpleasant distraction that sneaks into life. A few (yet too many in my opinion) of my clients and friends passed away at a very young age. When you devote your life to fitness, leaving this world in the early fifties doesn't seem right. That is only half way to reaching the potential of living to a hundred. I was baffled and started thinking more and more about Life and the power of the body and mind with respect to healing. Another direction in my personal and professional research began to take its course.

What is the healthiest way of living while focusing on performance and sports, taking in consideration the modern lifestyle that we live? What do we need to do to jump off the train of this modern lifestyle that is killing us prematurely?

"Simple" is the secret.

[3]

SIMPLE IS THE SECRET

For the past five years, I have been focusing more and more on the longevity and youthfulness in body and mind, while remaining productive in business and performing maximally in sports. During my research on what is best for health and longevity, I had to stay aware that we are athletes and we want to perform at the highest levels. Usually, maximum performance means extreme measures, which may not go hand in hand with health and longevity.

I have been looking at the new emerging population of high performing super athletes who chose plants for their main source of energy. Some call it vegan. I prefer to call it plant-powered or plant-based because that best describes it. The central part of your nutrition comes from plants, which means everything that grows under or above the ground, that doesn't have a face or a mother.

Healthy longevity and maximum performance is not an easy combination, but I have found an astonishingly simple solution: go back to the basics. Put aside the convenience of the modern lifestyle, look at what our grandparents were doing and adopt as much of it as possible:

1. Eat food as close to its natural state as possible: fruits, vegetables, legumes, grains, nuts, and seeds.

2. Prepare your food on your own so you have control over what you put into your body.

3. Get rid of all unhealthy non-necessities such as microwave ovens and bake, steam, or cook your foods instead. Even better, eat them raw.

Although our grandparents ate meat, poultry, fish, and dairy, there was virtually no mass production and the animals were healthy and nutrient dense. In our modern society, focusing more on production and consumption, we over-consume and get sick. We force-feed the animals with genetically modified foods and inject them with antibiotics so they can survive their unhealthy and already very short life span. The fish is farmed in unhealthy over-crowded pens. Then we transport them across the globe, wasting resources, so they can finally land on our plates, which are already too full. We are making ourselves sick and fat from over consumption.

If you cannot eat it, don't put it on your skin. The skin is the largest organ of the body and a powerful detoxifier. While it expels the bad stuff out of the body, it also takes in everything that we expose it to, bypassing the acids of the stomach, and going straight to the bloodstream and body. In a way, the result is much worse than if you ate the product. Look carefully at what you use on yourself. Our grandparents didn't use any fancy lotions, sunscreens, or fragrances. Next time you want to apply something to your skin, ask yourself "do I want to take a bite of this?" Use natural products instead, such as coconut oil, shea butter, neem oil, and similar items.

As I was looking more into the area of longevity and wellbeing, I was finding more disconcerting news and knowledge about the food processing industry. The fast food business correlates intimately to disease not just in America, but also across the globe as more countries are adopting this modern lifestyle. The lifestyle that is too busy producing and not caring about the health of the body and mind is slowly destroying people's health.

Just as in six degrees of separation, this is the first-degree of nutrition: go to the basics. Go directly to the source. There is no need for a middleman that processes the food into something else. You process your food with your own hands in your own kitchen. The food grows and you eat it. You are plant-based. You are powered by plants.

[4]

WHAT EATING STYLE IS BEST?

When people hear that I am a plant-powered athlete—I do look very fit, lean, and muscular—they look… then they think… they look more… and think. To make myself more clear, I say that it is kind of like a vegan. They immediately oppose me, stating that they crave meat, they love dairy, or they cannot cook without olive oil. And these are the "good" opponents, the healthy ones. I am not even talking about the fast-food-and-donut-with-cola, obese part of the population, which seems downright disconnected from what healthy nutrition means. The athletes usually get it.

Surprisingly, too many athletes eat unhealthfully. While only a small portion of athletes eats poorly by conscious decision, because they don't want to change their habits, the majority lacks accurate information and nutritional education. In this world of information overload, it takes much effort to sort through all the data to get a clear understanding of what is good and bad for us. Watching TV and reading mainstream fitness magazines doesn't do it. They just summarize an ongoing trend based on one study that may even be biased toward the funding company. That is why you hear that coffee is good, a few years later, it is bad for you, and after more time it is extremely good for you. Similar things happen with eggs, alcohol, carbohydrates, supplements, vitamins, and so on.

It takes a lot of reading of trustworthy sources and finding medical and health professionals who believe in the importance of nutrition. Then you have to analyze all the information, past and current, find scientific and anecdotal cases and put it all together. Understandably, only those with a keen interest to be healthy, energetic, and on peak performance will do this work, because it takes a lot of time and energy. You have to find it fun and motivating, or you won't do it. I did find it fun and motivating to do the research. Now you can benefit from my studies.

Maybe you have picked up this book because you are in search of the "right" kind of nutrition for improved performance. Perhaps you have just decided to become healthier, and this is your first step in making the transition, or you have been experimenting with many different nutrition styles and you are not sure if you have found the best one and are still searching.

I personally believe in the words that I write. I have strengthened this belief through my own experience and through several thousands of hours of researching what is the best approach, while communicating with other performance professionals and nutrition experts. There are many different opinions out there, sometimes completely opposing, sometimes they differ only slightly.

It is not easy to find the "right" way, because, after all, we are all different. It takes time to search and a lot of experimenting to practice. I believe that you will know when you find what is best for you during the final fine-tuning: you will feel great, have boundless amounts of energy, perform much better, and recover faster. You lose weight if you need to lose some and it happens in a simple and non-forceful way. You do not have any cravings; you eat to your satisfaction and everything on your plate looks and tastes exciting. The majority of your medical issues clear up. When you have this feeling, you know that you have found what is best for you.

The whole foods plant-based style of eating works for recreational athletes and elite or professional athletes in various sports: endurance, extreme endurance, contact sports, ball sports, or strength sports. Sometimes you encounter people who say, "I tried this vegan stuff, and it didn't work at all; I didn't have any energy, and I got sick." While I understand that it can happen, the solution is simple: eat more! Most of the time, this is the secret. Eating plants adds so much volume to your plate that you feel full before you get all the calories that you need. The stories of people who "wasted" away just confirm that they didn't eat enough. The harder you train and expend more calories, the more starches you need to add to your diet, because the colored vegetables and fruits just won't do it. Add the whole foods starches, legumes and small amounts of nuts and seeds and you will have all the energy you need.

Listen to your body, it will always tell you what it needs. If you feel that your skin is drier than usual, add more fat in the form of nuts, seeds, or avocados. If you feel tired, eat larger amounts of starches for carbohydrates and legumes for protein. If you are losing weight too fast, add foods that are more compact: starchy vegetables, nuts, seeds, and legumes. If you are gaining weight, take away the compact foods and eat more volume: fibrous vegetables and fruits. It is that simple. Don't blame the diet. Be pro-active.

Contemplating the plant-based lifestyle, you have probably encountered other nutritional styles that have become popular the last few years such as Paleolithic diet by Walter L. Voegtlin or the Perfect Health Diet by Paul Jaminem. They both focus on eating as our ancestors ate. They believe that our ancestors were meat eaters and they recommend eating meats and oils.

They are somewhat mistaken about the history of the hunter-gatherer, according to the highly prominent anthropologist Nathalien Dolomy Ph.D. who has explained in his various publications that our predecessors were mainly starch eaters. If they were meat eaters, their teeth and face would have developed differently, just like dogs and cats, for example.

Nevertheless, the foundation of the Paleo diets is good: they take away all processed foods and sugars and focus on some vegetables and fruits. Unfortunately, they allow eating meat, poultry, eggs, and oils, while restricting grains and legumes, and completely forbidding wheat and gluten. Often people fall in love with Paleo-style nutrition because they are not willing to give up animal products for emotional reasons, and the permission of animal product is like a security blanket.

There have been many discussions, both on respectful levels and in brutal verbal wars, trying to decide which is better: Paleo or whole foods plant-based nutrition. While this is not a finished conversation, I think we need to take personal responsibility and figure out which one is better for us. Try the Paleo for a month and pay attention how you feel and perform. Then try the plant-based style for a month and observe again. I am confident that you will feel the best while eating whole foods plant-based nutrition, if you are able to detach emotionally from the addiction to animal products.

I am very familiar with the plant-based diet—it has been my focus of interest for a long time, and I truly enjoy it and believe in it. Therefore, I will elaborate more in detail about this style, give you tips and the do's and don'ts so you can enjoy this healthy lifestyle fully, if you choose so. From my personal experience, I find the plant-based nutrition much easier and simpler than any other nutritional approach, and I have tried nearly all of them.

The simplicity of the whole foods plant-based diet is so beautiful: no animal products. That's it. No thinking about if the cow is healthy or not, fatty or lean, grass-fed or toxic from drugs. Your grocery shopping happens in the outer perimeter of your local store (have you noticed that all veggies and fruits are far out there?) or at local farmers markets. You can grow some in your garden as well.

Plant-based nutrition opens an unknown world of cool vegetables and grains that you may have never tried before. Feel free to experiment, and you will be pleasantly surprised as I was. If these are not enough positives, you will also find that eating plants is significantly less costly than eating animal products, especially when you have to choose the grass-fed, free-range, non-toxic animals. Once you decide in your mind that you can let go of your attachment to animal products, you will be the happiest plant-based athlete.

[5]

PLANT-BASED VS. VEGAN

Does eating whole plants mean that you are a vegan? This is a very sensitive subject, often talked about. If you look up the word vegan in the American Heritage dictionary, you get this definition:

> "A vegetarian who eats plant products only, especially one who uses no products derived from animals, as fur or leather."

Already here we may have a problem for many people. Many adopt a plant-based diet for the health benefits, yet they enjoy using animal products such as having a nice leather jacket or car seats. Often the word vegan is activist-like and people associate vegans with protest for animal rights and similar. While it is not necessarily true, not too many people know that and they usually judge vegans as a cult and attach other misconceptions. Many vegans care for animals and sustainable living and they passionately fight for it. They may care more about animals than about their own health, as eating vegan foods doesn't necessarily mean eating healthfully.

Vegans don't eat any animal products and often are so firm in their opinion that they say they wouldn't eat an animal product even if they were starving to death and didn't have anything else to eat. I am sure that I would eat anything in that situation, plant or animal. Plant-based athletes might consider the many health benefits of honey, whereas vegans consider honey an animal product.

Another problem with "vegan" is that it doesn't necessarily entail a healthy diet. There is so much junk vegan food, such as processed non-animal products, over cooked and under nourished meals, full of oil and other unhealthy additives. Eating fatty vegan sausages doesn't mean that you will become healthy.

In summary, the word vegan implies more than just plant-based dietary choices, reaching other, non-nutritional areas while it doesn't effectively express the healthy plant-based style of eating. I want to distinguish eating for optimal health, longevity, and maximum performance, therefore I call it plant-powered, or even more descriptively: whole foods plant-based nutrition.

[6]

MOTIVATION TO BECOME PLANT-BASED

We are lucky to live in this civilization of knowledge and information, as we have the luxury of knowing the leading causes of death. We have to use this information wisely and proactively work on halting, reversing, or even better, never getting heart disease. The easy way to do this is through nutrition, because you have total control over what you put in your body and over the outcome of your efforts. Don't rely on the excellent hands of surgeons to get you out of trouble later in life, rather, take the responsibility into your hands now.

Being fit from the outside is fine, but work actively on being healthy from the inside. The knowledge that you can prevent and even reverse heart disease is extremely empowering. Without a strong and healthy heart, your life and athletic prowess get complicated. Even though you can keep on living, the quality of life is not the same. You never will reach your maximum athletic potential. Taking care of your cardiovascular system should be the number one priority. If you don't have any signs of heart disease yet, you will never get it if you adopt a whole foods plant-based diet. If you have heart issues already, you need to be much stricter with your diet, but you will become healthy again. Scientists now understand relatively clearly what causes a disease, but unfortunately, these facts are not known by the public or even worse, by many physicians. While there are many amazingly skilled physicians in their fields, only a few have expertise in nutrition and its healing powers.

To understand better why nutrition has such a big impact on your health, let us look under the hood, or under the skin. The human blood vessels are coated with one layer of endothelial cells, which produce an essential gas called nitric oxide. This is almost a "miracle" gas. It widens the blood vessels so the blood can flow smoothly without sticking, and thus prevents the development of blockages. It also destroys inflammation. Because athletes and inflammation go hand in hand, nitric oxide is your best friend. You should always keep it in your mind when you make your food choices. Eating oils, dairy products, and meats will weaken the function of the endothelial cells, and eventually damage them. This will ultimately lead to vascular disease. Carefully constructed experiments show that even one meal of meat, oils, or dairy disables the endothelial cells from releasing nitric oxide for up to six to eight hours. Now imagine meal after meal, day after day. The damage is enormous. For maximum athletic performance, you want to keep your arteries as clean as possible.

While all scientists agree on the connection between nutrition and disease, the opinions on therapy are conflicted and often contradicted. Imagine that you are served a toxic ingredient that would make you extremely sick instantly. You would probably not think twice whether or not to eat it, right? Now, when you have the precious knowledge that meat, oils, and dairy injure your body from the inside, albeit very slowly and over a long time, wouldn't it be a good decision to abstain from these foods?

Dr. Caldwell Esselstyn successfully helped many terminally ill patients, who committed to turning their health and life around with the help of nutrition. This approach is inexpensive, quick, long lasting, and you have command of the situation.

Even though you may not currently have any signs of cardiovascular disease, there are things happening on the inside that we don't see and feel. For an athlete, even a slightly compromised cardiovascular system will reduce the maximum performance and ability to train hard and recover properly. If health and longevity are not strong enough motivation, the training capacity and performance is a reflection on what is happening inside you. Nutrition needs to be your number one priority. Commit to it and you won't regret it.

[7]

TRANSITION

While you are transitioning to a whole foods plant-based diet, you will need a little extra discipline and focus in the beginning, because you may feel an emotional loss when you stop eating your favorite animal foods. You will look for something else to fill that empty space. You may worry about getting hunger attacks and intense cravings.

However, you will realize very quickly how extremely easy it is to get used to the delicious and satisfying starches, vegetables, and fruits instead of heavy, rich, and often chemically enhanced animal products. But, until this happens, you will need a little discipline to stick to your new nutritional style, just as in any other change or transformation.

CHANGE IS UNCOMFORTABLE

Change is not always easy, whether you choose it consciously, or it happens because of circumstances. It can be uncomfortable or downright painful. That is why we fear change. Even though we are consciously choosing health and vitality, for some people the idea of never eating meat and dairy can still be horrifying. Others may take it on with ease. We are all different. Easy or not, remember that this significant change doesn't need to happen overnight. This is going to be your new lifestyle and you can ease into it and feel comfortable.

FIND A METHOD THAT WORKS FOR YOU

Maybe give up meat and dairy just for one day a week (there is already a support organization called Meatless Monday). You will find that it is actually rather simple. Then you may add another day or two and string a few days in a row. Finally, perhaps you may do six meatless days a week and have one meaty one. One day, you will have all days without meat and dairy because you feel great.

Some people need to quit cold turkey because it is too difficult for them to eat just a little bit of the animal products, teasing their taste buds constantly. Remember that there are no rules. Do whatever best fits your personality and lifestyle.

The change is progressive. Even though you don't eat meat and dairy, there will be moments where you are passing by your favorite restaurant or you smell your friend's lunch and your memories bring the temptations and a tiny drool to your mouth. You may succumb, especially during the first stages of your transition. Don't worry, enjoy your meal and keep going. It's not the end of the world.

As time goes by and you feel healthy and thriving, it will be harder to tempt you. You will know when you are one hundred percent plant-based—when no image of animal products, TV commercial, or smell will arouse your taste buds or your mind. You will be unmoved, and there will be no temptation to taste a piece. You may even reach a point where you see a juicy cheesy hamburger on TV, and your face will scrunch, thinking, "Ewww; that's nasty!" If you are laughing in disbelief now, remember these words for the future.

TRANSITION

In the beginning, you may find potatoes, rice, lentils, beans, or grains a bit bland compared to your previous rich animal meals. I promise that it won't take too long and you will truly appreciate their taste. In next to no time, you will never want to look back at the animal products again.

During the transition, if you need to enhance your carbohydrates with something that your taste buds are accustomed to, such as BBQ sauce, mustard, ketchup, vinaigrette, spices, or sweetener, please do so. It is better to add something familiar rather than drift off the path. After all, you were always adding these condiments on your meats, didn't you? Meat without spices is rather boring.

It may come as a surprise that I am suggesting sweeteners. Unprocessed sweeteners, such as honey, agave syrup, maple syrup, or molasses are fine to use. While they all contain sugar, it is a safe and clean source of energy without added fat, sodium, cholesterol, or other chemicals. You need to use it smartly and sparingly and it will be a great addition to your culinary expedition to plant-based heaven. Stevia (the plant Stevia rebaudiana, also known as sweet leaf) is a safe sweetener to use without adding extra calories.

Sugar is a much better choice to enhance the flavor of your food rather than fats and oils, which hold twice as many calories per gram and a collection of medical problems associated with it. No need to worry, as the sugar in your plant-based kitchen will not make you fat or diabetic.

Some studies suggest that people who eat more simple sugars ingest fewer total calories and thus have less of a chance of becoming overweight. The mechanism is that they feel satisfied faster with the sweet flavor, and consequently eat less fat. Type-2 diabetes is a result of obesity. The lowest rates of obesity are found in nations where high-carbohydrate diets are the cultural style of eating, for example in rural Asia, Africa, rural Mexico, or Peru. When these people move to modern areas and adopt the fatty and processed Western diet, they become fat and sick, despite their "genetic make-up". The genes play a very small role, while lifestyle dictates almost all outcomes in life. Scientists understand that sugar doesn't cause type-2 diabetes and the American Diabetic Association recommends that diabetics eat 55–65 percent of their daily calories from carbohydrates. Whole foods plant-based nutrition helps diabetics cure their conditions, reduce, or completely stop their medications and improve their overall health and wellbeing.

Whether your style of transition is gradual or instantaneous, if you have a hard time, you can make the transition easier by using vegan substitutes for your favorite animal foods. Even though I do not recommend them for your future nutrition, I think it is ok for short periods if it simplifies your transition. They are usually highly processed with various additives, and your goal is to transition away from man-made food to whole plants in their natural state.

All this said, it doesn't mean that you can binge and adopt a diet full of processed, white sugar and flour, sugary donuts, and other processed carbohydrate foods. If the food doesn't grow above or below the ground, it is processed, and you don't eat it. The food processing takes away all the quality nutrients, and the refined foods are nutritionally empty. Even if they enrich the processed foods with some other "good" nutritional ingredients, most often, they are chemically created and the body doesn't know how to process or use them. In your new plant-based life, this is not food.

PROCESSED VEGAN FOOD

Some of these substitutes look, smell, and taste like their animal cousins: soy burgers and sausages with painted grill marks, tofu pieces looking like chicken, pizza with fake mozzarella cheese made from soy. They make your life easier during the transition, but try to eat them minimally and for only a short term. Processed soy products, often drenched in vegetable oils are as bad as animal products. Modern food processing factories use fast and mechanical methods to turn soy into edible copies of other foods. Many of the processing methods are unsafe and health threatening as described in detail by Dr. John Briffa in his article *It's not just the salt that makes many meat-substitute foods a thoroughly unhealthy option:*

> "The food industry has contrived to contrive soya into a huge range of processed foods by converting raw soya beans into something known as soy protein isolate (SPI). Production of SPI takes place in factories where a slurry of soybeans is treated with acid and alkali solutions to get the protein to precipitate out. In this process, the product can be tainted with the metal aluminum (aluminum exposure has been linked with an increased risk of degeneration of the nervous system and Alzheimer's disease). The resultant protein-rich 'curd' is spray dried at high temperature to produce a powder. SPI may then be heated and extruded under pressure to make a foodstuff known as textured vegetable protein (TVP). SPI and TVP will usually have monosodium glutamate (MSG) added to it to impart a 'meaty' flavor before it is fashioned into products such as vegetarian burgers, sausages and mince."

Even though you are still doing a great thing—saving the lives of poor animals—you are not doing a good thing for yourself. Once you are deeper into your transition, you will discover many yummy foods to eat, with a chewing consistency that gives you the same pleasure as animal products. You will discover that you don't need any substitutes for your favorite animal anymore because you will create your own meals such as a great burger from lentils or garbanzo beans, a cheese-like spread from cashews or white beans, or tasty desserts from beans and seeds. Your creativity will bring joy to your meals and health to your life.

[8]

COST OF BECOMING VEGAN

When people think of organic vegetables and fruits, they think, "It's too expensive." On the contrary, you will find that transitioning to plant-based nutrition will cost less, and depending on your sources, can be significantly less.

If you buy your plants when they are in season, the prices will be very low. Farmers' markets have affordable prices of local, organic produce. I understand that different places in the world have better or worse possibilities of getting plentiful variety of organic produce, but when you put in a little effort, it is possible to find farmers' markets almost everywhere.

Years ago, I used to have an aversion to Whole Foods Market because of their high prices. I felt that I couldn't afford to spend all my money on food. Over time, as I was getting deeper into learning about the health benefits of fresh, organic, and non-GMO produce, I have realized that it is a tiny price to pay for being healthy, energetic, and thriving.

During the years of my personal research and training, the organic movement has shifted for the better for us customers. When I later revisited my neighborhood's huge, recently built Whole Foods Market to buy one small thing, I was pleasantly surprised to find prices that were so much better than I remembered. I couldn't stop exploring, observing and desiring almost everything in their huge selection. While it is true that organic still costs more than conventional, the difference is getting smaller.

Let us look at the prices. A meat eater needs to take into consideration that the conventionally and industrially produced meat and poultry are loaded with toxins, chemicals, and antibiotics and thus she should be eating grass-fed cows and free-range birds. The prices of these products are quite high: over $10 per pound of beef, $15 for a pound of fish, and $8 for a pound of organic free-range chicken. Organic milk costs approximately about $4 per gallon, organic cheese costs $10 per pound, and organic yogurt costs $4 per quart. Statistically, an average person eats about a half pound of meat and one pound of dairy a day, which can cost $10–$15 a day. However, a typical carnivore eats higher than average amounts.

You can get two pounds of organic broccoli, two pounds of organic fruits, five pounds of organic carrots, and five pounds of organic potatoes for $10–$15 per day. This does not even mention how many pounds of organic rice, quinoa, or oatmeal you could get. Putting this into perspective, eating organic whole food plant-based nutrition is not as expensive as we tend to think. I have made comparisons of costs for meat eaters, fish eaters, vegetarians, and vegans just to get an idea. The total costs vary for different states and cities, but the relative differences remain similar across the country.

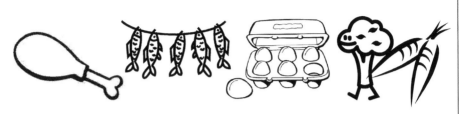

	Meat-Eater	Fish-Eater	Vegetarian	Vegan
Breakfast	Wheat toast ($0.25)	Wheat toast ($0.25)	Wheat toast ($0.25)	Oatmeal ($0.30)
	Bacon, 3 strips ($1.60)	Smoked salmon	Yogurt, 1 cup ($0.80)	Blueberries ($0.80)
	Egg, 1 piece ($0.20)	1 oz ($1.30)	Blueberries ($0.80)	Orange juice ($0.40)
	Orange juice ($0.40)	Orange juice ($0.40)	Orange juice ($0.40)	
	Total $2.45	**Total $1.95**	**Total $2.25**	**Total $1.50**
Lunch	Turkey sandwich with	Tuna sandwich with cheddar cheese	Tomato, mozzarella, pesto sandwich	Hummus, red pepper, tomato sandwich
	Swiss cheese ($2.20)	($1.95)	($1.70)	($1.70)
	Carrots ($0.30)	Carrots ($0.30)	Carrots ($0.30)	Carrots ($0.30)
	Apple ($0.90)	Apple ($0.90)	Apple ($0.90)	Apple ($0.90)
	Total $3.40	**Total $3.15**	**Total $2.90**	**Total $2.90**
Dinner	Chicken fajita ($7.30)	Fish fajita ($7.80)	Tofu fajita ($5.80)	Tofu fajita ($5.80)
	Taco cheese ($0.35)	Taco cheese ($0.35)	Taco cheese ($0.35)	Guacamole ($0.45)
	Sour cream ($0.20)	Sour cream ($0.20)	Sour cream ($0.20)	Side salad ($0.50)
	Guacamole ($0.45)	Guacamole ($0.45)	Guacamole ($0.45)	
	Side salad ($0.50)	Side salad ($0.50)	Side salad ($0.50)	
	Total $8.80	**Total $8.40**	**Total $7.30**	**Total $6.75**
All Meals	**$14.65 Meat-Eater**	**$13.50 Fish-Eater**	**$12.45 Vegetarian**	**$11.15 Vegan**

The data and my personal investigation suggest that the meat-eating lifestyle costs the most, while the vegan lifestyle is the cheapest. While some people believe that veganism is a lifestyle choice for hippies and rich materialists, this is not true. I do believe that it is very hip to care about your body and health, with a magnificent side effect of rescuing many animal lives, and preventing the destruction of nature and natural resources, but it is definitely not rich and materialistic living. It is the opposite: living of awareness and caring.

Generally, the plant-based sources of protein (legumes, tofu, and seeds) are much less costly than the meat-derived versions. While it is possible to be an expensive plant-based eater and a low-budget meat eater, looking at the average, the plant-based regimen wins over the meat eating one, and the fish eaters and vegetarians float around in the middle. Plant eaters can save up over $10 dollars per day, which means savings thousands per year.

Processed foods are the foes in any well-balanced diet. They are very unhealthy and very expensive. Vegan and vegetarian processed products, such as Tofurkey, vegan meatballs, soy hot dogs, or prepackaged non-meat burgers, can raise any budget because they may be even more expensive than the animal-based processed products. Stay away from all processed foods to the best of your ability.

Grains, starchy vegetables, and legumes are highly cost-effective, especially when you buy in bulk. When you make them staples of your plant-based nutrition, they deliver high amounts of calories and protein at a much lower cost than animal products, even when you add the slightly more expensive, fresh, organic vegetables and fruits to your starches.

People often argue that organic produce is extremely expensive and has no evident advantage over the conventional produce. This is not fully correct, but you can think about it like this: organic is like the private school of food; if you can afford it and if you can find it close by you, go for it. Don't panic if you cannot eat organic; eating conventional produce has more benefits to your health than not eating it at all.

Eating in restaurants is not just highly costly but it is also relatively unhealthy. Even when you have good intentions and choose a "healthy" meal, you never know what is going on behind the kitchen curtains such as how much extra oil, sugar, or other flavorings has been added to make the food taste delicious. Now you pay a lot of money for something that is not very safe for you. The estimations suggest that one in three Americans eats at fast-food restaurants daily. While it may appear that it is much cheaper to eat in a fast food place, it is still much more costly than eating at home. And we are just considering the price of the meal, not the price of your destroyed health.

The amount of money spent on food correlates directly to how much money people have. In 2009, people making $40,000 to $50,000 a year spent $5,560 on food. People earning more than $125,000 spent $12,655. People spend about 10% of their yearly income on food. The wealthier people don't eat more food, but they buy more expensive foods such as better cuts of meat, more organic foods, and more prepared or gourmet foods. They pay extra for the convenience and the quality. On average, people spend approximately 60% of their food cost on eating at home, and slightly above 40% of total food cost on eating out.

2,500-CALORIE COST EXAMPLE

A moderately active man consumes about 2,500–3,000 calories, and a moderately active woman consumes 2,000–2,500 calories per day. Let us look at the various foods and their cost per 2,500 calories.

The following calculations don't reflect everybody's situation exactly, of course. The prices vary in different cities, states, and the world's countries, so consider the following numbers with an open mind. However, the calculations do reflect the main conclusion: the whole foods plant-based life style is much cheaper than the modern animal product diet.

The prices are calculated for 2,500 calories, based on price per pound. The prices are for conventional products. Grass-fed beef and free-range chicken cost much more:

Animal Food	Cost per 2,500 cal	Cost per item	
Salmon	$30.60	$9.99	/lb
Beef rib eye	$24.29	$9.99	/lb
Cheddar cheese	$15.48	$11.99	/lb
Chicken breast	$13.72	$3.99	/lb
Milk	$10.37	$4.99	/lb
Ground beef	$6.55	$2.99	/lb

People eat at fast food restaurants for two reasons: they feel like they don't have time to cook at home and they think that fast food is much cheaper. While it sounds cheap looking at the menu, when re-calculated per 2,500 calories, it is not that cheap. The cost of your destroyed health, doctor visits, and medicine is not included, and it will add multiples of the cost in the future. I list a few basic fast food items to present the average cost and to reveal the misconceptions of fast foods' low cost.

Surprisingly, the prices of the "cheap" fast food are quite high, ranging between $11 and $20 for 2,500 calories. The quality of fast food is terrible, and you pay a high price now and an even higher price when you get sick in the future.

Fast Food		Cost per 2,500 cal	Cost per	item
McDonald's	Chicken Sandwich	$20.77	$3.49	/item
Subway	$5 6-inch Special	$20.00	$5.00	/item
KFC	Oven Roasted Twister	$19.10	$3.19	/item
Taco Bell	Chicken Salad	$17.06	$5.39	/item
Round Table	Ulti-Meat Pizza	$14.83	$21.35	/item
McDonald's	Big Mac	$14.77	$3.19	/item
Taco Bell	Taco	$14.56	$0.99	/item
Burger King	Chicken Sandwich	$12.62	$3.99	/item
Burger King	Whopper	$11.12	$2.99	/item

Consuming legumes, grains, and starchy vegetables is a different story. Since they don't spoil easily, you can purchase them in bulk for a much better price. Even with the grains, legumes, and starchy vegetables, if we choose to buy organic, the prices go up, but for comparison to the cost of animal products, this example is sufficient.

Plant-based Starchy Food	Cost per 2,500 cal	Cost per	item
Sweet potatoes	$3.00	$5.99	/10 lbs
White potatoes	$1.75	$6.99	/20 lbs
Brown rice	$1.52	$24.75	/25 lbs
Oats	$1.05	$6.99	/9 lbs
Pinto beans	$1.05	$13.79	/25 lbs
White rice	$0.44	$14.99	/50 lbs

Adding fresh, perishable vegetables and fruits to the menu will increase the cost, just as it will by adding them into the meat eater's menu. Adding two pounds of veggies and fruits will add another $3–$4, increasing the total per 2,500 calories

		Calories	Carbs (g)	Fat (g)	Protein (g)	Chol (mg)	Potass (mg)	Cost
Early AM								
Coconut Creamer (So Delic.)	3 tbs	30	3	0	0	0	0	$0.10
Coffee	8 oz	5	0	0	0	0	232	$0.40
Raw organic Manuka honey	1 tbs	70	18	0	1	0	0	$0.30
		105	**21**	**0**	**1**	**0**	**232**	**$0.80**
Breakfast								
Bananas raw	120 g	107	27	0	1	0	430	$0.30
Kale raw	70 g	35	7	0	2	0	313	$0.40
Pineapple bits (frozen)	3/4 c	70	19	0	1	0	150	$0.65
Hemp seeds raw organic	30 g	170	3	13	10	0	0	$0.60
		382	**56**	**13**	**14**	**0**	**893**	**$1.95**
Lunch								
Walnuts (Kirkland's)	30 g	200	4	20	5	0	125	$0.50
Coconut milk kefir (so Delic.)	2 c	140	12	12	2	0	0	$2.00
Blueberries wild, frozen	420 g	240	57	0	3	0	225	$3.00
		580	**73**	**32**	**10**	**0**	**350**	**$5.50**
PM Snack								
Spirulina organic (nuts.com)	1 oz	80	8	2	16	0	0	$0.80
Corn thins (Real Foods)	8 pc	176	32	0	4	0	0	$0.60
Raw organic Manuka honey	2 tbs	140	36	0	0	0	0	$0.30
		396	**76**	**2**	**20**	**0**	**0**	**$1.70**
Dinner								
Red beets raw	300 g	135	29	1	5	0	975	$1.60
Potato raw	800 g	616	140	1	16	0	3,368	$0.80
cucumber raw	200 g	30	7	0	1	0	294	$1.60
		781	**176**	**2**	**22**	**0**	**4,637**	**$4.00**
Eve Snack								
Raisins seedless sun dried	20 g	65	16	0	1	0	0	$0.20
Light coconut milk (TJ's)	80 ml	50	4	4	0	0	0	$0.10
Carrots raw	350 g	144	34	1	3	0	1,120	$0.30
		259	**54**	**5**	**4**	**0**	**1,120**	**$0.60**
TOTALS		**2503**	**456**	**54**	**71**	**0**	**7,232**	**$14.55**
		Calories	Carbs	Fat	Protein	Chol	Potass	Cost

My calorie proportions of carbohydrate to fat to protein were approximately 80–10–10. I do not follow any particular ratios of the macronutrient proportions, but I do make sure that I follow the suggestions and philosophies of my favorite nutrition experts, doctors, and specialists as often as possible.

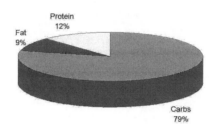

Dr. Esselstyn recommends keeping the fat around 10–15% from calories and Dr. Campbell recommends keeping the protein between 8–12%.

Other outstanding lifestyle and nutrition specialists include Dr. Joel Fuhrman, Dr. Dean Ornish, Dr. Neal Barnard, Dr. John McDougall, Jeff Novick, Dr. Michael Greger, and Dr. Michael Klaper.

While my fat intake is a bit on the lower side in this example, it usually varies between 10–15% and on occasions up to 20–25%. My protein intake is between 8–15%, depending on the food choices that I make for that specific day. On the days when I eat more legumes, I may achieve higher levels of protein. In the example above, I eat a lot of organic fresh produce, which is usually assumed to be too expensive, yet my daily cost is still cheaper than eating fast food. On the days when I eat more legumes and grains, the cost decreases dramatically toward the numbers of the grain-eating person in the previous section.

The total cost of one day of fresh, mostly organic produce in my example above is just under $15, which is just as much as eating processed, fattening, and disease-creating fast food in the previous calculations.

There is no reason to choose fast food over nutritious and healing whole foods!

[9]

IMPORTANCE OF FOOD FOR HEALTH AND PERFORMANCE

Staying healthy and fit appears to be more complicated than it should be. Even though there are many factors involved, not too many people understand the power of food in healing and performance. The majority of people don't realize how important food choices are for their health even though they all know that health is critical to performance. They don't correlate what they eat to how sick they have become and that with better decisions they would thrive in health and energy.

According to the science, approximately 70% of deaths in North America and about 65% in the entire world are directly connected to the lifestyle and the food that we eat. Experts estimate that almost all diseases are entirely preventable by diet and lifestyle changes, up to 90% for type-2 diabetes, over 80% for heart disease, and at least 60–70% for cancers. People who already have the disease can stop it and even reverse it by eating less and excluding all processed foods.

The evolution of "real" food into processed food has been the biggest disaster in our health history and completely detrimental to our health. The food industries take healthy food, from which they remove everything that has nutritional value and all the natural flavors that we like such as sugar, fat, and salt in their natural form. Instead, they add a mixture of chemical junk to make the foods look better. Then they add large doses of chemically processed sugar, fat, and salt that are scientifically created to reach the bliss point, to make them taste even more addicting. This nutritionally empty and highly addictive, calorie-laden junk food is the worst thing that has happened to our health.

There is no justification for anybody to eat this way. We have the possibilities and resources to eat fresh, nutritious food, but we need to re-learn how to eat in the ways in which our grandparents used to eat. We need to educate ourselves as to what is best for us and not just blindly trust the medical system and doctors, unless they are experts in nutrition and longevity. Only a very few medical professionals are trained in nutrition, but hopefully this will change soon, because we do have a medical crisis. Our medical system is set up to treat people's symptoms with drugs and surgeries. While this can be useful at times, it is not useful for treating chronic disease and creating lifelong health. People need to change their lifestyle by exercising more, eating less, and choosing nutritious foods.

The fast food and junk food industries sponsor many of the national food campaigns. Just because you see tempting foods on TV doesn't mean that they are good for you. It is difficult to know what is healthy for us and what is not because we are constantly bombarded with wrong and often contradicting messages. Ultimately, it is on us to educate ourselves and find the truth. You have taken the first step by picking up this book, and hopefully it will deliver more understanding of your new nutrition lifestyle, improved health, longevity, and maximum athletic performance.

Often you hear that eating bad foods, fried foods, or processed foods is okay as long as you do it in moderation. This message only feeds your emotions and your fears. It delivers what you want to hear because in the beginning it feels scary to think that you "will never eat that pizza again." These fears make you dislike every message that suggests that eating meat and dairy is bad for you. You would rather hear that moderation is okay. Moderation is not okay. Moderation kills. Fried processed foods are bad for you and every meal that you eat including these items is making your health worse. Seventy percent of the population is dying from diseases that are results of eating these foods. There is no moderation in being dead. It may seem harsh, but that is the message that we need to hear over and over to take this matter seriously, because it is extremely serious.

Smoking was enormously popular up until the mid 60s (in 1964, the United States Surgeon General's report on Smoking and Health came out, suggesting a link between smoking and cancer), and nobody believed it could be bad, because the cigarette companies were denying any health risks. We fought, and we won. This will eventually happen with our food supply. More medical professionals, dieticians, and other health care professionals are aware of the critical situation of our food system and the medical crisis. They are starting to spread the words of awareness. It will take some time, but it has begun and we all can do our part in the development that is for the best for all of us, including our health, happiness, and longevity. As a great side effect, we will get a better environment, less animal cruelty, and better economy. All these issues are intimately interlaced.

REAL LIFE CHOLESTEROL EXPERIMENT

I had been a vegetarian for quite some time when a chain of events occurred. First, I saw the movie *Forks Over Knives* and was extremely impressed with its message and even more with the expert presenters. They were radiant, healthy, and energetic even at an older age. What a true inspiration! They motivated me to pick up their books and learn everything they have to share.

I started with *Prevent and Reverse Heart Disease: The Revolutionary, Scientifically Proven, Nutrition-Based Cure* by Dr. Caldwell Esselstyn. His message and theories were so convincing that I immediately booked an appointment to get my blood work and cholesterol levels checked. Because I live a healthy lifestyle, exercise regularly, and eat vegetarian foods, I believed that my numbers would be impeccable, but I was curious if the numbers were what Dr. Esselstyn stated that they should be. According to the standard measures, I was doing great, but the standard was not good enough for me. My new standard was Dr. Esselstyn's suggestion: total cholesterol below 150 mm/dL.

Description		My numbers	Normal
Total cholesterol	mg/dL	171	100–199
	mmol/L	4.42	2.59–5.15
HDL (good cholesterol)	mg/dL	56	> 36
	mmol/L	1.45	> 0.93
LDL (bad cholesterol)	mg/dL	115	0–99
	mmol/L	2.97	0–2.56
Total triglycerides	mg/dL	100	0–149
	mmol/L	1.13	0–1.69

That day, I decided to become 100% plant-based. For the next three months, I became as extreme as Dr. Esselstyn suggests in his book. I would become an oil-free vegan. Let me see if he is right and my numbers get better. No processed oils were allowed, meaning no olive oil, no coconut oil, and no flax seed oil. Small amounts of nuts, flax seeds, hemp seeds, avocado, and other plant sources of fat were allowed, as long as the total daily intake of fat doesn't exceed 10–15% from calories. My past relationship with nuts was truly nutty: I loved them so much so that I could eat bags of them. No wonder my triglycerides were on the high end.

At the end of this 3-month experiment, I went to get my blood drawn again. The results were truly impressive. Considering that I was already rather healthy before the experiment started and it is much harder to improve something that is already quite good, Dr. Esselstyn theories proved right. Everything improved considerably.

Description		My numbers	Change
Total cholesterol	mg/dL	147	-24
	mmol/L	3.8	-0.62
HDL (good cholesterol)	mg/dL	53	-3
	mmol/L	1.38	-0.7
LDL (bad cholesterol)	mg/dL	82	-33
	mmol/L	2.12	-0.85
Total triglycerides	mg/dL	61	-39
	mmol/L	0.69	-0.44

I must conclude that this experiment was a great success. The wisdom of eating plants and plant-based nutrition demonstrates the benefits. My energy levels were consistent and surprisingly high after drinking the green smoothies. My weight has been stable at my optimal, lean weight of 160 lbs. The most exciting experience of these three months was the amounts of food that I could eat. I love to eat and the volumes were plentiful, while the calories were not excessive. For people who love to eat, eating plants is the way to go. Eat until you cannot eat anymore, minding your fats, and you still won't gain any excess weight.

[10]

IS THIS LIFESTYLE FOR EVERYONE?

Reading and comparing all the positives and negatives makes it obvious that the whole foods plant-based diet is one of the better things we can do for ourselves. It will bring great results to any person of any age and any fitness level. Even though it makes perfect sense, not everybody will turn to plants to improve their health and performance. Today's views on health and nutrition are indoctrinated and driven by the false social and economical forces that create more disease and problems than ever in our history. It is hard for people to change their beliefs and habits. People would rather age prematurely, live their lives in pain and obesity, and die too early, than challenge their beliefs and change their lifestyle.

I wish, but I do not expect, that everybody will want to change and adopt this healthy lifestyle. Many people remain trapped in their current destructive habits, such as smoking, too much alcohol, stress, and too many unhealthy foods. We all have an individual journey, and we reach certain points at different speeds and from different directions.

I am grateful that you have picked up this book and are considering turning your life toward health, wellbeing, and maximum athletic performance.

SECTION 2

BASIC NUTRIENTS and FOODS YOU CAN EAT

[11]

PROTEIN

In my bodybuilding career, I was stuffing myself with protein from early morning to late night, regularly eating 250–350 grams a day. When getting ready for a competition and cutting the carbohydrates dramatically (yes, we used to believe that carbohydrates made you fat), I had to eat even more protein to get my calories from something other than fat. As I was changing my lifestyle and eating smaller amounts of protein, I was feeling better and lighter.

Yes, I did lose some body weight when I started to play tennis, but it was partially because I was running on the court for hours every day. It is hard on the body to be heavy while running around on the concrete, when you need to be quick, agile, and explosive with the endurance to do this for hours. My weight dropped 20 pounds and adjusted at 160 pounds, where it has stayed ever since. With body fat levels at 11–15%, this is a fine result for an almost half-centurion plant-eating woman. This result is convincing enough that plant-based nutrition is sufficient, healthy, and great for maximum performance.

So what is the truth about protein? How much protein do we really need? From my personal experience, while trying all possible protein amounts, I need to say that plant-based nutrition delivers enough: enough of the quantity, enough of the quality. Yet another great result of the simplicity of the whole foods plant-based diet is that you get enough for your health and performance and not too much to get sick and slow. Personally, I eat about 80–140 grams per day, which is about 10–15% of total calories. These are great numbers. You don't want to eat much more, as you will discover in the following pages.

For the last two centuries, the protein recommendations have been swaying from one extreme of super high protein diets to another extreme of very low protein. The debate is still going on, even as there is more evidence that high protein is harmful to your health. The high protein proponents (and I used to be one of them) may make the body look beautiful from the outside, chiseled and lean, but it is not looking or feeling good deep inside. Studies are confirming that adequate protein intakes from plant-based nutrition are the healthiest for your body and its longevity and vitality. Improved performance is what you get as the cherry on top of your cream. Oops, there is no cream in your plant-based diet.

Is plant protein as good as animal protein and dairy? When I tell people that I am plant powered, they look at me in disbelief at first. I look too strong and meaty and don't fit their image of a typical vegan. They think of vegans as scrawny, sickly, non-radiant skinny people. But here I am, all tanned, strong, and powerful. What is wrong with that picture? When nothing is wrong, they tell me that they just love meat too much. They cannot imagine their life without meat.

When I suggest that meat doesn't really taste so good, they start fighting me. Have you ever tried to eat your meat plain, without any spices, salt, sugar, fat, sauces, and other additives? It is actually really bland and boring. It is not the meat that tastes so great, but all the combination of spices that you marinate it in before preparation. If the spices do the job, why can't you use them for your plants and make them taste completely as yummy? Just don't say that the meat is delicious.

Meat, poultry, fish, and dairy all contain a lot of protein, fat, cholesterol, and dietary acids, while they almost never provide any healthy fiber. When we eat more than our body can metabolize, neutralize, or exert, the excess will convert into substances which are toxic to our bodies, and their effect is cumulative over time. The acid weakens the bones and the fat and cholesterol clogs the arteries. The elimination process of excess protein overloads the liver and kidneys.

There is a link between animal products and our modern chronic diseases such as cancer, heart disease, diabetes, and many other problems. It doesn't matter if the animal product is processed or cleanly produced by a local farmer. The amounts that we typically consume in our modern western society will slowly create disease in the body.

Unfortunately, the misconceptions about our protein needs are enormous. Protein is one of the most provocative and the least understood food topics. The meat and dairy industry have a strong political and financial power, influencing the norms and guidelines of dietary needs. They scare people with the dangers of not drinking enough milk for your bones or not eating enough quality protein, which you only get from animals, as they recommend. People fear getting sick from too little protein, while they are not noticing that they are getting sick from too much protein. I challenge you to think of one person that has died from a lack of protein, while many lives have vanished due to diseases from excess protein.

Dr. T. Colin Campbell suggests that there is a strong correlation between dietary protein intake and cancer of the breast, prostate, pancreas, and colon. The higher the protein intake, the higher rates of cancer there are. In his research, when they lowered protein intake to 5% of total calories, the cancer rates went down, not so mysteriously. When they raised the protein intake again, the cancer rates went up. In addition to cancer, excessive protein intake causes constipation and other digestive disorders, autoimmune disorders, arthritis, osteoporosis, premature aging, impaired liver function, kidney failure, and heart disease.

Too much protein puts extreme physiological stress on the body so that its healing process is disrupted, which creates ideal conditions for chronic diseases. It is nearly impossible to find adults who don't have any of the chronic conditions. A completely healthy adult person is more a phenomenon than normality.

There are several studies, current and past, which confirm that a daily intake of 5–10% of calories from protein is optimal. The 5% intake is sufficient, so you have room to play with if you consume 5–10%. The average American eats 15–16% of calories from protein, and on many occasions even more, up to 20–30%, as is often seen in strength athletes, people who want to lose weight by eliminating carbohydrates, and many other populations who fear not getting enough protein.

HOW DOES EXCESS PROTEIN CREATE DISEASE?

One explanation is that the excess protein clogs the basement membranes in the cells, which perform the necessary job of filtering the oxygen and nutrients into the cells, and the waste products out of the cells. When the basement membranes are clogged, the good stuff (nutrients and oxygen) cannot get in and the bad stuff (waste products) stays trapped inside the cells, which causes low oxygen levels and malnutrition in the cells, decreasing the pH of the bodily fluids to levels low enough to cause illness. Animal protein is mostly acidic, while the body wants to be slightly alkaline.

When you eat too many acidic foods, the body immediately works on neutralizing the acids to create its balance again, by leaching alkalizing minerals such as calcium from the bones and teeth. Excess protein cannot be stored in the body so the kidneys will work on eliminating it. It puts extra strain on the kidneys, which over time can cause diminished function or kidney disease. Luckily, this is reversible, so converting to low fat, low protein plant-based nutrition will help your kidneys to restore their power.

There is a difference between animal and plant-based protein. While there is a misconception that animal protein is superior to plant protein, it is not as correct as the meat and dairy industries claim. It is true that animal proteins have the most similar amino acid profile (the building blocks of protein) to the human protein and therefore are highly efficient when used for synthesizing the human protein.

However, this does not mean that animal protein is best for us—the opposite is true. Just like pushing the gas pedal to the floor, accelerating the synthesis makes many other functions accelerate as well, causing premature aging, heart disease, diabetes, osteoporosis, and cancer. In the race of life, the secret is going slow. The plant proteins (inappropriately named the "low-quality" by a mistake that has been later admitted, but this misconception is now too well spread) allow for slow and steady synthesis of new proteins, which is much healthier for us. They are incorrectly labeled as low quality because they don't come as a "complete" package in terms of matching our protein make-up as a group.

Nevertheless, they contain all of the proteins that we need to thrive and be healthy. By eating a variety of plants, we receive all the amino acids needed to feel great, while minimizing the risks related to eating animal proteins. The plant proteins do what the animal protein does, but with greater effects, especially when talking about athletic performance and muscle building.

Many high-performance athletes are plant powered: Dave Scott, the six-time winner of the Ironman triathlete; Carl Lewis, the seven- time gold medalist Olympian sprinter; Rich Roll, the multiple Ultraman champion and one of the fittest men in the world at age 45; Martina Navratilova, Serena and Venus Williams, 75-year old bodybuilder Jim Morris, strength athlete Mike Mahler, bodybuilder Robert Cheeke, Mixed Martial Arts champion Mac Danzing, ultra-endurance athletes Brendan Brazier and Scott Jurek, and many more. The list of these plant-powered amazing athletes is too long to be listed here. They train, compete, and thrive on plant-based diet with impressive results and health.

Our nation's health is at its lowest, while the consumption of animal products is at its highest. People start searching for different ways, and many find the answer in plant-based nutrition. They heal their chronic disease, slow down or reverse aging, improve performance, and achieve tremendous health overall. I have personally witnessed many of my clients and fellow tennis players, who followed my path into the world of plants improving their health, losing weight to optimal levels, reducing and eventually eliminating their medications, and performing at their best. Even the most hard-headed meat lovers admitted humbly that there is something unique about plant-based nutrition.

PROTEIN AND ELITE ATHLETIC PERFORMANCE

Protein sources are labeled as complete and incomplete according to how many essential amino acids they provide. A complete protein provides all of the essential amino acids. Animal products such as meat, fish, poultry, eggs, and dairy are considered a complete protein and sometimes called a "high quality" protein. Such unfortunate labeling brings various deep-rooted misconceptions. On the other hand, an incomplete protein lacks at least one of the essential amino acids, but combined together they provide sufficient amounts of the essential amino acids. For example, rice combined with beans or mixed varieties of plants provide all the vital amino acids.

The human body assimilates an animal protein much easier because it is more similar to the human protein, and some athletes and bodybuilders find this appealing because they think they will grow their muscle tissues faster. However, just as the muscles grow faster, all the other cells reproduce and multiply much faster, and this can be dangerous when cancerous cells find an environment promoting fast growth. The plant protein is absorbed less efficiently than animal protein, but it is more beneficial for humans.

The Minimum Daily Requirements (MDR), now called Estimated Average Requirements (EAR) are the minimal requirements for the body to function. They are calculated from the amount of lost nitrogen that needs to be refilled by consuming protein. Decades of scientific research have determined that the minimum requirements are about 5% of daily calorie intake, which is approximately 0.5–0.6 g/kg or 0.23–0.27 g/lb. For a 160-pound person, the minimum daily requirement is 36–44 grams of protein. The modern westerner gets this amount in one meal

The Recommended Daily Allowance (RDA) was set in 1943 through reliable, scientific experimentation and it is reviewed every five years. Each time, it stands the test of time. If we eat a whole food, plant-based diet, the protein we consume is the equivalent to the RDA. The RDA takes into consideration special populations with special needs and widens the limit to about 8–10% of daily calories, which corresponds to 0.8–1.0 g/kg or 0.36–0.45 g/lb. These amounts ensure that 98% of people will meet or exceed their physical needs. For a 160-pound person, the recommended daily allowance is 58–73 grams. Eating whole foods plant-based nutrition delivers nearly perfect amounts of protein, about 8–10% of calories.

The popular belief is that athletes require higher amounts of protein for optimal performance, and strength and power development. It is more common among strength athletes and bodybuilders, but even endurance athletes believe in heightened amounts of protein for a proper recovery.

Athletes easily ingest 1 gram of protein per pound of bodyweight, and that is usually the lower limit of their range. Bodybuilders eat up to two or more grams of protein per pound of bodyweight. I know it myself. As a drug-free bodybuilder, I always believed that I needed extreme amounts of protein to grow muscles and to remain lean. I ate about 40–50 grams per meal (which is just above the minimum daily allowance) and I ate 5–6 such meals every day, which totaled nearly 200–250 grams of protein per day, approximately 40% of total daily calories.

Other common nutritional approaches among athletes were 40–40–20 (40% calories from protein, 40% from fat, 20% from carbohydrates), or even more extreme low carbohydrate diets with only 10% of calories from carbohydrates, and the rest was protein (30%) and fat (60%). Dr. Atkins was the promoter of his high-fat and high-protein diet, which years later was revealed to have created many severe health problems.

In the early 2000s, increasingly more athletes started to look for a better way to get an athletic edge. If you compare elite athletes, they all train hard and the physical preparation looks quite similar. So how does one separate from the rest? The answer is the recovery. If everybody prepares in a similar way, then the recovery will make a difference. If you recover faster and better, you can train harder and more intensely.

There are several things that you can do to promote optimal recovery, and while they were just experimental and "weird" at the end of 1990s, they are now part of standard training regimen: stretching, massage, myofascial release, sauna, and other techniques such as yoga, meditation and visualization or hypnosis. Everybody is looking for that extra edge. While everybody is looking, it is surprising that more athletes haven't touched on the subject of nutrition. The trend is starting slowly, but one would think it would be more widespread. There are power athletes, martial artists, ultra endurance athletes, and others who have entered the world of fine-tuning their nutrition for maximum potential.

Many professional athletes, world-class elite athletes, and even passionate fitness enthusiasts usually assume that more protein is better, and that large amounts of protein will give them more muscles and better athletic performance. Why do athletes have these beliefs? Why did I used to believe it?

The father of nutrition and mentor of many nutrition experts of today, Carl Voit (1836 to 1908) believed that 52 grams of protein a day is the requirement for a "man." Already then, there were discussions about protein and they continue to this day. To make the picture clear, Russell Henry Chittenden (1856–1943) created an experiment with himself and his student subjects. He put them on a low protein diet (below 50 grams a day) and tested them in 15 endurance and strength exercise tests from October through April. To everybody's surprise, the students doubled their performance! The critics of Mr. Chittenden were suggesting that the students would do even better if they were on a high protein diet. So he created another study with students who already were at high, world-class fitness levels. He switched them from high protein to low protein diets and retested their fitness levels after six months. He got results that are even more remarkable: the group of students that was already at world-class fitness levels improved about 30%. Astonishing results!

While bodybuilders and strength athletes eat excessive amounts of protein, the majority of which is excreted in the urine (expensive pee-pee), if you ask dancers or endurance athletes, they often cringe at a photo of a juicy steak. Somewhere in between, there is a happy "meat-ium." We need the protein to build and repair muscle and tendon tissues, fingernails, hair, red blood cells, and to synthesize hormones and enzymes. Protein is necessary to improve healing and recovery.

PROTEIN REQUIREMENTS

According to Nancy Clark's *Sport Nutrition Guidebook*, a sedentary adult needs 0.4 grams of protein per pound of body mass; an active adult needs 0.4–0.6 grams per pound, a growing athlete 0.6–0.9 grams, and an adult who is building muscle mass requires 0.6–0.9 grams per pound. If you are a 160-pound tennis player, you need 96 grams of protein per day, which is about 384 calories. On a 3,500-calorie diet, it corresponds to 9% of calories. 3,500 calories per day may sound high, but that is what I eat as a female tennis player. You will notice that you will be able to eat more food after transitioning to whole foods plant-based nutrition. If you love food and eating a lot, this is great news.

Example of a 160-pound (72.7 kg) adult			
	g/kg of body weight	g/lb of body weight	g/day for a 160 lb person
RDA	0.8–1.0	0.36–0.45	58–72
Sedentary adult*	0.9	0.4	64
Active adult*	0.9–1.3	0.4–0.6	64–96
Growing athlete*	1.3–2.0	0.6–0.9	96–144
Muscle-building adult*	1.3–2.0	0.6–0.9	96–144
*according to Nancy Clark's *Sport Nutrition Guidebook*			

The recommended daily values and the *Sport Nutrition Guidebook* recommendations are just what they are: recommendations. While these are great baselines, you need to develop a good relationship with your body and adjust your needs according to the present status of your body's demands. Generally, 90–95% people shouldn't eat more protein because they are already constipated from eating too much protein and eating more of it will make things worse. Even more important than how much protein you eat is how much protein your body extracts and assimilates from the foods. It depends on the health of your digestive tract. Keeping your digestive tract healthy and efficient will reduce the amounts of protein you need to ingest, because you will be able to assimilate almost all of it. Individuality is extremely broad, so nobody can really tell you how much, and what YOU need. A few markers of your protein status are:

1. You need to eat more protein if you experience fatigue, reduced recovery from exercise, muscle and joint aches, emotional depression, sleep disturbances, hormonal imbalances, or loss of sex drive.

2. You need to eat less protein when you have smelly sweat, smelly urine and feces, and when you bowel movement doesn't flow. In addition, your breath may be stinky.

Follow the personal indicators of your protein needs, which will depend on your lifestyle, health, and activities. Keep monitoring your energy levels, exercise recovery ability, mental clarity, sleep quality, sexual performance, and overall state of happiness. Protein requirements can be higher during periods of illness or recovery.

Protein intakes within 10–15% of total calories greatly fulfill all athletes' needs; even athletes who want to increase muscle mass fit well into this range. For the muscle-growing athletes the total calorie intake is more important than the protein intake. If sufficient calories and carbohydrates are delivered, the body uses the protein for building muscle mass rather than for energy. If the athlete wants to lose weight or body fat and therefore eats fewer calories, then the protein needs may be higher, up to 20% of total calories.

For whole foods plant-based athletes, it is necessary to eat a variety of plants to get the full spectrum of amino acids. Those athletes who choose not to eat processed protein sources such as tofu, soy shakes, or vegan cheeses and sausages, may encounter a reduced digestibility of whole food plants and may need to eat 10–15% more protein. This is very personal and I recommend experimenting with different amounts while observing the performance and recovery. Generally, eating a variety of whole food plants delivers enough protein and no extra protein powders are necessary.

	g/kg of body weight	g/lb of body weight	g/day for a 160 lb person
Example of a 160-pound (72.7 kg) athlete			
Standard training	1–1.2	0.46–0.55	73–87
Endurance training	1.2–1.7	0.55–0.77	87–124
Power/speed	1.2–2	0.55–0.91	87–145
Early stages of muscle building	2–2.3	0.91–1.05	145–167

The typical "more is better" is not true when you are talking about protein. That's why it is necessary to experiment to figure out the optimal range for your personal athletic needs. Eating excessive amounts of protein won't improve athletic performance nor increase muscle mass. It can be dangerous to your health and performance. One misconception about excess protein in your diet is that it can cause kidney damage. While it cannot cause kidney damage, it makes the kidneys work harder.

Another problem is that excess protein is converted to fat and stored or used for energy by oxidation. Protein oxidation creates a byproduct that needs to be excreted in urine, which increases the risk of dehydration. For the cost-conscious person, protein costs much more than carbohydrates and using protein for energy becomes unnecessarily expensive.

There is a chance of getting too much protein mainly if you supplement your whole food plant-based diet with protein powders, protein bars, and other processed protein sources. If you rely entirely on plants, you are safe and don't need to worry about eating excessive protein. The only time to use supplemental protein is if you don't meet your caloric demands, or if you travel and have difficulties finding good sources of whole food plants. Sometimes you may not have time to cook or create a whole foods meal, and then a quick protein bar or protein smoothie will come handy.

DAIRY MISCONCEPTIONS

You need to drink milk to get strong bones, right? Yes, you can get calcium from eating dairy products; however, it is not your best option. Actually, it is a bad decision. Even though we hear from early childhood how important it is to drink milk to get strong bones and teeth, it is more myth than truth.

Calcium is an essential mineral for all living beings. The majority (99% of it) is stored in the bones, and its purpose is to build a strong skeleton, and to regulate the functions of the nervous system and blood vessels. In nature, mineral comes from the soil and the growing plants absorb the calcium through their roots into their leaves. Cows eat the grass and transfer the calcium to the milk that we drink. But is it really so efficient to use the cow and her milk as a medium of the calcium transfer? Why not get it straight from the source: the plants? In addition to a lot of calcium, there are various other minerals in the vegetables and fruits.

We don't need to worry how to get our calcium, rather how to retain it in our bodies. In the human body, the gastrointestinal tract, the bones, and the kidneys precisely regulate the calcium balance. If you eat too much calcium, the body gets rid of the excess, and if you eat too little of it, the gastrointestinal track works hard to extract more of it from the foods, while the kidneys preserve what is in the body. Calcium deficiency is unknown in people eating a natural whole foods diet.

Many studies suggest that the countries and populations consuming the highest amounts of milk and other dairy (United States, Canada, Sweden, Norway, Australia, New Zealand) have the highest rates of osteoporosis and hip fractures. Consumption of milk and dairy actually harms our bones. The most dangerous foods are the ones containing a lot of animal protein and dietary acids such as meat, poultry, hard cheeses, and fish. When you eat high acidic foods, your body attempts to neutralize its environment by pulling the calcium from the bones. Over time, the bones will become brittle. Eating plants, which are alkaline forming, is a much healthier alternative to supply the body with calcium together with other beneficial healthy nutrients.

The majority of dairy products contain a lot of fat. Eating dairy in excess makes people sick and overweight. Calcium supplements are not recommended because they disturb the balance of other minerals. Eating a variety of plants will deliver enough calcium even for the hardest training athlete.

Simply put, dairy is bad. It carries a lot of infectious agents, viruses, bacteria, and other harmful elements. Milk is as bad as meat, usually much worse for one important reason: sometimes we are aware that too much meat is not good for us, but the saying "milk is good for you" is imprinted in our minds since early childhood, and many people believe that milk is super healthy.

If you are willing to change just one thing on your journey to health and optimal performance, you should eliminate dairy first. You will be surprised how great you will feel. If you have allergies, they will dissipate. If you have digestive issues, they will be gone and with them many other physical ailments that we usually don't consciously link to eating dairy.

DAIRY SUBSTITUTES

For me, giving up meat was not as difficult because I was not eating it very often. I was too lazy to prepare it at home, and I was not eating in the restaurants often. However, eliminating dairy seemed like an impossible task. I really loved Greek yogurt, which with the frozen berries tasted like a delicious ice cream. My Slavic roots insisted on drinking several glasses of kefir (fermented dairy beverage) daily. I also enjoyed adding heavy cream to my morning coffee. Without the cream, I didn't even care to drink the coffee. The heavy cream made my coffee and my day to start right. I also had a few favorite light cheeses. See, I used to be a relatively big dairy consumer. Now, I have to give up all this? Becoming dairy-free was the hardest step during my transition. However, once I made up my mind and systematically went to figure out the technicalities, this was the best thing out of many that I have accomplished during my dietary transformation.

There are many companies producing delicious non-dairy milks, yogurts, creams, and ice creams, using coconut milk, almonds, soy, rice, and more. It is extremely simple to make your own non-dairy milk using almonds, walnuts, pecans, cashews, oats, or rice.

NUT OR GRAIN MILK

Use one cup of nuts of your choice and soak them overnight. Add 3 cups of water and blend in a blender. High performance blenders such as Vitamix or Blendtec will do an amazing job; other blenders are functional too. Blend until smooth. Some nuts such as almonds will produce a grainy consistency that you should strain through a strainer or a cloth. You can use the pulp for baking. Other nuts such as cashews create super creamy consistency without the need for straining.

When using grains, such as rice, oats, barley, rye, cook the grain first, and then proceed as when using nuts. Uncooked and soaked oats deliver a slightly different essence to your milk.

If you want flavored milk, add one or more of vanilla, cocoa, maple syrup, cinnamon, nutmeg, or anything that you like. To make thick milk, with a creamy texture, reduce the amount of water to half or to your liking.

To create your own cultured beverage or yogurt, add lemon juice to the milk or cream. The milks can be stored in the refrigerator for several days. Use them in smoothies, cereal, cooking, baking, or make your own healthy ice cream mixed with frozen fruits.

CHEESES AND SPREADS

Even after adjusting to using my homemade milks, I continued to miss the texture of light cheese on my bread. A homemade spread is a great substitute for cheeses. Take a can of white beans and blend them in the blender. Add a tiny amount of lemon juice and spices to your liking, such as pepper, garlic, or salt, and blend until smooth. Use the spread on the bread, for dipping or wrapped in a tortilla. Adding nutritional yeast will create a cheesy flavor. For different variations of spreads, use black beans, garbanzo beans, lentils, peas, or edamame.

[12]

CARBOHYDRATES

The best carbohydrates for your health and performance are complex carbohydrates—even though they are not as complex as they may seem, but rather quite simple—brown rice, whole oats, white, yellow, red, and other potatoes, sweet potatoes or yams, corn, and other grains. If you can, choose organic or non-GMO approved, so you are on the safe side of the GMO conflict. One day, hopefully we will win this war and have only clean healthy foods around us, but until then we need to be more conscious and choose organic if possible.

GLYCEMIC INDEX

If you have ever followed any diet regimen of high-fat or high-protein diets, you are very familiar with the "evil" glycemic index, aka GI. If you haven't, you are one of the few, because it is nearly impossible to avoid it. Glycemic index measures how much the blood sugar rises after eating different foods. The high-fat or high-protein diets make you believe that the higher the GI, the worse the food is for you and that you should not eat any of the yummy high GI foods, such as jasmine rice, boiled potato, carrots, brown rice, baked potato, and others, because they will make you fat and sick. On the contrary, the increase of disease and type-2 diabetes is enormous when people exchange healthy carbohydrates from plants for low-GI, fatty foods like meats, cheeses, and vegetable oils.

The rise of your blood sugar after a meal is actually a good thing. That is the reason we eat in the first place—to get all the nutrition quickly in and into the blood stream. Why should we be so scared of that? After eating a meal, the blood sugar goes up, peaking above 130 mg/dl within 40–60 minutes for the high-GI foods, while for the low-GI foods it takes about 90 minutes to peak at 100 mg/dl. The rising blood sugar creates feelings of satiety, telling your brain that you should stop eating now, rather than continue eating excessively and gain weight. Calorie per calorie, potatoes satisfy your appetite twofold compared to meat or cheese. Potatoes have a high glycemic index.

ATHLETES AND GLYCEMIC INDEX

Athletes use high-GI foods to quickly replenish the glycogen levels lost during their performance or to carbo-load before the completion or race. Any athlete will benefit from full glycogen stores, giving them energy for high performance. Even if you are not an athlete, but you want to be strong and energetic, the starchy carbohydrate will be your best friend. Don't be scared of the high-GI healthy foods. If you choose your foods according to the blemished reputation of high-GI foods, you may make terrible mistakes. Pizzas full of cheese with dripping fat or fatty hamburgers have much lower GI than boiled potatoes, carrots, or plain rice. There is no need to explain which one is healthier. Everything can be very misleading sometimes.

If you are one with a strong sweet tooth, this entire chapter is probably making you very excited. While I defend the high glycemic carbohydrates and sugars to a point, I need to declare a warning: eating high amounts of simple sugars is not good for you. It will elevate the blood triglycerides levels and create tooth cavities. Eating beyond the point of being full, almost to a discomfort level (which could occur with simple sugars) will force the liver to turn some of the excess sugar into triglycerides. Heightened levels of fat in the blood lead to an increased risk of heart disease and stroke. Don't be scared of carbohydrates, though. When you eat whole grains, beans, and potatoes, accompanied with some green and colored vegetables and don't overstuff yourself, your triglyceride levels will be fine.

If you already have elevated cholesterol and triglycerides levels, this whole foods plant-based eating style will normalize all your numbers relatively quickly. If you are one of the few whose numbers don't go down as much, even though your energy and wellbeing have dramatically improved, you may need to eliminate all refined flours and simple sugars, including fruits and juices. Fructose, the sugar found in fruits, has a tendency to increase the triglycerides the most. If you don't have any health issues, you don't need to shy away from simple sugars and fruits, just don't overdo it regularly.

CARBOHYDRATES AND ELITE ATHLETIC PERFORMANCE

Today, the science of training and peak performance is so advanced that it seems almost impossible to get that extra edge. Nutrition is one of the roads less traveled and an increasing number of athletes are discovering the importance of nutrition. Whether you are a weekend warrior or an elite athlete, you will maximize your potential through nutrition when you find the right balance of energy and nutrients.

The energy that fuels your performance comes from glucose and fatty acids. Depending on your fitness levels and the activity's duration, intensity, and type, different energy sources are utilized, aerobically or anaerobically. The aerobic metabolism uses oxygen (the primary fuels are fatty acids, and small amounts of glucose) and is predominantly used in distance running, biking, swimming and similar activities. The anaerobic metabolism happens without oxygen as it doesn't completely metabolize glucose, which creates residues of lactic acids that cause the burning sensation in the muscles and fatigue. It happens during the first moments of an intense activity during sprinting, bursts of energy in ball sports, wrestling, and weight lifting. Both energy systems are essential.

Eating a whole foods plant-based diet may increase energy requirements by 10–15% because of the reduced digestibility of the high-fiber foods. For weekend warriors, who exercise only a few times per week, the energy increase may not be significant, but serious athletes who train hard daily may need 3,000–6,000 calories a day. Many athletes strive for low body fat levels and keep an eye on their energy intake. If you lack energy regularly, you most probably don't eat enough calories. Eating too little can harm your performance by decreasing your metabolism and thus not having enough energy available for training. You can play with your calorie intake and increase it by up to 500–1,000 calories and see if that will improve your performance without harming your body fat levels.

A daily intake of 3000–6000 calories of plant-based whole foods may sound like a tremendous volume of food. Yes, it is! If you have difficulties eating large volumes of food, include more dense foods such as nuts, seeds, nut butters, and homemade baked goods.

Carbohydrates are the preferred source of energy for athletes, and an inadequate intake of carbohydrates will harm optimal performance. The American and Canadian Dietetic Associations recommend a diet of 65–70% of calories coming from carbohydrates for adult athletes; the fat recommendations are in the 15–20% range. Way back in 1968, the research suggested (and has never been disproved) that a high-carbohydrate diet might increase the athlete's endurance threefold through allowing maximum glycogen stores: the athlete can work with greater intensity for longer periods before fatigue sets in. The glycogen lasts for about 90–120 minutes of work at intensities of 60–80% of VO2 max (maximal oxygen consumption). At higher intensities, the glycogen lasts a much shorter time. Proper endurance training increases the glycogen storing capacity of muscles, but to be able to use it to the maximum, you must provide high amounts of carbohydrates, approximately 6–8 grams per one kilogram, which is 2.7–3.6 grams per one pound of bodyweight. An athlete weighing 160 pounds needs to supply the body with 430–580 grams of carbohydrates, which corresponds to 1,700–2,300 calories per day from carbohydrates.

Another benefit of whole foods plant-based nutrition is that it supplies abundant amounts of carbohydrates necessary for training and peak performance. Whole grains, vegetables, and fruits are excellent carbohydrates. In combination with legumes, nuts, and seeds, they deliver large quantities of vitamins, minerals, and phytochemicals, which are all extremely important for maximum performance.

While sugars and refined carbohydrates are technically carbohydrates as well, they don't supply any additional nutritional value, and you should restrict their intake to about 10% of the total calories. The newer guidelines by American Heart Association and some other nutrition experts are even stricter: they recommend no more than 5% of your total calories from sugars.

If you consume 3,000 calories per day, allow only 150–300 calories or less from plain sugars, which equals approximately 37–75 grams, or 2.5–5 tablespoons. It sounds like a lot, but one 20-oz bottle of Gatorade or soda contains 34 grams of sugars. The majority of people drink more than one bottle. I do not suggest drinking sugary sodas, however. Drink plain water, and if desired add a bit of honey, blackstrap molasses, or maple syrup.

GRAINS

There are many different opinions regarding grains. Some are valid, and others are just plain myth. People often fear grains and think of them as "an evil starch" that will make them fat. The truth is that the processed grains (and processed foods) will make you fat, but you shouldn't fear whole grains. Nowadays, people are not capable of recognizing a whole-wheat berry, buckwheat, barley, rye, millet, or brown rice because they only eat processed forms of white breads, quick oatmeal, white rice, grits, cornmeal, and other highly processed cereals.

Ancient people cultivated grains for thousands of years, understanding their nutritional value for human development, vitality, and prevention of disease. Grains combined with other whole foods include all the elements needed for health, longevity, and performance.

Once you achieve healthy levels of digestion—and eating whole foods makes this happen fast—the grains will satisfy your hunger and taste without any unnecessary cravings, they will provide you with energy and endurance, calm nerves, quick reflexes, clear thinking, improved elimination, and deep sleep.

Compared to processed grains, whole grains require slightly different preparation for proper digestion. You also need to chew them differently for the salivary glands to work correctly: chew them really well, up to thirty times or more. Sick people who need to extract even more nutrients and whose digestion may be weaker, should chew each mouthful fifty or more times. This is very unusual in our fast-paced world with meals in a hurry, usually swallowed on the run, and fast food eaten in the car. Nonetheless, this little change of eating slowly and chewing deliberately will bring great results to your digestion and your inner peace. This chewing technique applies to other fibrous foods such as legumes, nuts, seeds, some vegetable stems, roots, and leaves.

Whole grains and some other carbohydrates don't digest properly without extensive mixing with saliva. Saliva's enzyme, ptyalin, changes carbohydrates into maltose. The enzyme maltase in the intestines breaks down maltose into the simple sugar dextrose and that is the end of the process. The enzyme maltase can only break down maltose and maltose can be only created with prolonged chewing. Otherwise, other processes such as unhealthy fermentation will occur. Saliva is alkaline, and while whole grains are mildly acid forming, a thorough chewing will make eating grains more alkaline and health-promoting.

Whole grains, legumes, and vegetables are called complex carbohydrates. Complex carbohydrates are an important component in healthy nutrition. Ironically, they are the most deficient element in the modern western diet, having been replaced with fast foods and highly refined and nutrient-deficient grains and sugars. Eating refined carbohydrates causes a sugar rush followed by a crash with instant cravings and depression. Complex carbohydrates offer a steady, balanced, and harmonious metabolism, delivering many essential nutrients. You will be surprised how filling and satisfying the complex carbohydrates are. You will feel an abundance of energy and drop any excess weight you may carry.

For maximum benefits of eating grains, follow these simple steps for proper preparation:

1. Wash the grains gently and soak them for eight to twelve hours. Soaking the grains will germinate the dormant energy, release the nutrients, and make them more digestible.

2. Discard the soak water and use it for watering your plants, as there are many nutrients in it. Fill the pot with fresh water. Different grains require different amounts of water. Generally, for one cup of grains, use three to five cups of water. If you have larger amounts of grains, reduce the water amounts or cook longer.

3. Add ¼ teaspoon or less salt for one cup of grains. One cup of grains serves two average people or one hard training athlete. I eat the entire cup myself.

4. Roasting grains will make them more alkaline.

5. Cooking the grains on low heat (below 200 degrees) will make them more alkaline and preserve many enzymes. Cook 30–60 minutes. Some grains may need longer time.

6. Remove the grains from the pot after cooking because they tend to expand and "sweat". When they become damp, they lose their taste. Blend them before serving so all the layers mix together.

7. Either serve or store them in a cool place for later use in salads and other meals. If they ferment a little bit, they will be more digestible and sweeter, however too much fermentation will make them inedible.

Increase your nutritional repertoire by experimenting with a variety of different grains to create exciting meals with amaranth, barley, buckwheat, kasha (roasted buckwheat), corn, millet, oats, quinoa, rice, rye, wheat, spelt, and kamut.

WHEAT AND GLUTEN

Wheat dominates our modern nutrition. Unfortunately, the majority of it is processed or genetically modified. Compared to other grains, wheat absorbs a wider range of nutrients from the soil. While this is healing and growth promoting (do not eat it in excess if you need to lose weight), wheat frequently promotes allergic reactions, particularly when ingesting flour that is rancid from oxidation. Wheat flour should be used *immediately* after grinding. Many allergic people are only allergic to the processed flour and can safely eat pre-soaked and cooked whole berries, sprouted wheat, or wheat germ. If you develop digestive problems such as bloating, gas, or pain, you should probably not eat wheat. For years, wheat has been considered an ideal food for growth, but since people are overeating rancid wheat products that are also genetically altered, they are now experiencing various sensitivities, allergies, and severe health issues.

Second only to sugar, gluten is the most prevalent substance in the modern western diet. Gluten is a solid, elastic protein that remains after washing all starch away from wheat flour. You can see the rubbery strands when you knead the dough to make bread. Gluten makes up 80% of protein in grains of wheat, rye, and barley. In some individuals, gluten may be toxic to the intestinal tract by altering the cell membrane structure, reducing the gut surface area, and thus impairing digestion. The single layer of the intestinal tract has two functions: it has to allow the food proteins and other nutrients into the body, and the opposite function of prohibiting parasites, viruses, and bacteria to enter the body.

The immune system is efficient in clearing all the gluten from the gastrointestinal tract, but in sensitive individuals, this process can cause inflammation in the intestine or stomach. In people with celiac disease, this single layer of cells is destroyed entirely, causing a condition called leaky gut, where alien proteins from microbes and foods can enter the body through the damaged intestinal wall and cause various problems. People with untreated celiac disease suffer from autoimmune diseases, such as type-1 diabetes, thyroiditis, psoriasis, lupus, lymphoma, and others, and may die prematurely.

About 50–60% of people are intolerant or sensitive to gluten. For athletes, gluten sensitivity has a serious impact on performance. Gastrointestinal tract inflammation causes muscle inhibition because they are on the same neurological channels and the gluten sensitive athlete is plagued by musculoskeletal problems that will not go away.

Some people have a heightened sensitivity to gluten: 30% can develop antibodies against gluten locally in the gastrointestinal tract and 11% systemically, which can cause additional problems in the future. Only a few individuals, about 0.4% of the population, will develop celiac disease where the immune system attacks and kills the gut cells and damages the intestine to the point that the person cannot absorb nutrients from foods.

The only treatment of celiac disease is through a diet that is low or free of gluten for the rest of your life. You need discipline and motivation to stick to this regimen. The positive news is that the intestine will heal, the leaky gut will stop leaking, and the malabsorption of nutrients will vanish. You will regain your health again.

There are no good tests to figure out the levels of sensitivity to gluten. One effective way is to eliminate all gluten products from your diet for two to three weeks, and then slowly bring them back. Feel how your body responds. If you don't feel any difference, you are doing fine. If you feel a stronger response, you may be more sensitive, and you should either completely stop eating processed wheat, or decrease the amounts to avoid discomfort. Proper preparation, such as sprouting and cooking of wheat in its grain form (wheat berry), may eliminate many issues while allowing you to still enjoy the nutritional benefits of wheat.

Before doing your gluten experiment, make sure you have transitioned and settled into the plant-based nutrition lifestyle. First, get rid of all the bad, processed, or allergen foods, and eat a clean diet before you experiment with eliminating all gluten foods. Pasta, white breads, processed snacks, pizza dough, or cookies are technically plant-based foods, but contain processed flour, which is most probably aged and spoiled, and may create a reaction in your body. You should be avoiding processed foods anyway, so transitioning to a plant-based diet may reduce any symptoms that you have.

In recent years, increasingly more people are becoming sensitive to gluten, with symptoms ranging from very mild to severe. During your gluten-free test, you may notice a new feeling that you never knew was possible. Feeling much better without gluten is a sign of gluten sensitivity. You may choose not to eat gluten at all, or limit the amounts. In any case, while paying attention to gluten, you will realize how many food items contain gluten. Even though the grocery stores carry more gluten-free items these days, it is still not very easy to be gluten-free and you may find it challenging. Frequently, gluten is added to any food that needs to stick together such as breads, pastas, ketchup, vegan processed meat substitutes, and many more. It is highly advisable to avoid substitutes and processed foods entirely after you have successfully transitioned into a plant-based diet.

If you find yourself extremely sensitive to gluten, you should eliminate wheat pasta and use rice or spelt noodles instead. If you don't have any gluten sensitivity, your life is going to be a little bit easier, but you should not eat any processed grains, and always choose the whole grain version, which has more nutrition, vitamins, and enzymes. The best option is to sprout your grains to enhance the enzyme content, protein quality, essential fatty acids, and the vitamin content. Sprouting creates a healthier version of the grain. You can bake your own breads and bakery items from sprouted grains. If you don't like to bake, you can buy sprouted bread, "Ezekiel 4:9" by Food for Life. They carry many different flavors, and even tortillas that you can use for making delicious wraps.

GLUTEN-FREE DIET

Eliminate all foods containing gluten: barley, einkorn, emmer, kamut, rye, spelt, triticale, and wheat (durum and semolina, bulgur, seitan). When making sourdough bread, Lactobacilli bacteria will remove most of the gluten and make the wheat tolerable for the majority of sensitive people. Be aware that all beer, ales, and malted drinks contain considerable amounts of gluten.

Acceptable grains without gluten are amaranth, buckwheat (or kasha), corn, millet, quinoa, rice, sorghum, wild rice, and oats. Some people may not tolerate oats, but most will. Make sure that the oats are not contaminated with wheat from the processing factory.

Enjoy all root vegetables, such as potatoes, yams, sweet potatoes, and cassava-root (tapioca) that are safe, gluten-free, and deliver a steady bulk of calories for the hard training athlete. Additionally, consume all other vegetables of all colors, all fruits, and all legumes such as beans (including soy and garbanzo), peas, and lentils. Chew the legumes slowly and properly so you don't suffer from the extra gas that causes bloating and bowel discomfort, which often is confused with celiac disease symptoms.

The beauty of the whole foods plant-based diet is that it is healthy even for the most gluten-sensitive person as long as you avoid the few above-mentioned glutenous grains. The rest of the huge colorful kingdom of plants is there for you to gobble anytime and anywhere, producing great side effects of improved health and performance.

[13]

FAT

Fat contributes up to 75% or more of energy requirements during endurance training. As the primary source of energy, fat is a vital nutrient for athletes. While athletes often fear dietary fat because they think it will make them fat, they are not completely right. Even though fat can convert to body fat much more efficiently than carbohydrates or protein, it can only happen when the total calorie intake is excessive.

In the body, the extra fat is stored in several places: under the skin as "subcutaneous fat" that is the most obvious, around the organs as "visceral fat," and within the muscle as intramuscular fat (your muscle tissue is marbled), which is available instantly as fuel during exercise. Lower levels of physical activity may lead to excess skeletal muscle fat content, which is strongly associated with obesity, type-2 diabetes, and metabolic syndrome. During high intensity exercise, the intramuscular fat is used first, making your muscles look and feel firmer. Then when that fat is depleted, the subcutaneous fat will be used, creating a leaner looking physique.

The amounts of fat that we need to consume depend on the amounts of carbohydrate and protein. When eating 70% of calories from carbohydrates and 10–15% from protein, the fat will comprise the remaining 10–15% of energy. For a 3,000-calorie diet, the athlete consumes about 33–50 grams of fat.

The best sources of fat are nuts, seeds, avocados, and butters from seeds and nuts. While some experts do not recommend eating any oils, because they are processed and the nutritional density is low, many athletes choose to include some extra flaxseed, coconut, or olive oil. It mainly depends on your health and if you want to become completely oil-free.

In our Western society, coronary artery disease is the leading killer, while it is an unknown disease for four billion people worldwide. It is strictly a disease of the modern Western civilization. All the previously healthy cultures that have adopted the Western lifestyle suffer from it now as well. Americans consume 135 pounds of fat every year (four times more than recommended), and by the age of sixty, they have consumed over four tons of fats and oils. Almost everybody develops a vascular illness at some stage of his or her life. The chronically heightened levels of cholesterol and fat in the bloodstream will narrow and block the arteries.

Dr. William Roberts, an expert investigator of cardiovascular disease, has established that there is only one true risk factor in coronary artery disease: the lifetime cholesterol levels of over 150 mg/dl (3.88 mmol/L). Regardless of the genetics, family history, whether it is hypertension, obesity, smoking, being a male or female, or other risk factors, keeping the cholesterol levels below 150 mg/dl will not initiate or worsen atherosclerosis, and it practically makes you heart attack-proof. If the cholesterol levels rise above 150 mg/dl, the risk factors may accelerate the disease. Lowering the fat intake to 10–15% of total calories keeps the blood cholesterol under 150 mg/dl, according to Dr. Esselstyn and Dr. Ornish and their successful studies with many heart patients.

NUTS AND SEEDS

While nuts and seeds are known to be very healthy for you, we need to look at them from a slightly different angle. In nature, they grow in a shell, and it takes hard work to get the nut out when you want to eat it. In our modern lifestyle, the nuts come prepackaged, shelled, usually roasted, and salted. You don't need to exert any energy when you extract a nut from the bag into your mouth. A little handful of 180 calories and almost pure fat takes only a few second to eat. Sometimes you eat them aimlessly and ingest many hundreds of calories together with extreme amounts of fat for the body to process into energy.

When you eat too many calories, the large portion of ingested fat will be stored as fat in your gut and hips for the starvation times, which never come. You just get fat. Athletes don't need an excess of dead weight (metabolically inactive fat tissue) that will slow them down and drain their energy.

Trees produce nuts and plants produce seeds for storing energy when it is time to reproduce. They will sprout into a seedling that can grow into a plant. Nuts and seeds are very rich in fats (nearly 80% of calories and only 10% of carbohydrates). They contain many minerals, vitamins, proteins, and other essential nutrients needed for the growth of the seedling. They are ideal for creating the new plant life but not as perfect for us because of their high fat content. We can have a few handfuls of nuts and seeds a day, but usually we overindulge and create not just visual problems such as oily skin and fat body, but also diseases connected with obesity such as type-2 diabetes, cardiovascular disease, and degenerative arthritis of hips, knees, and other joints. A fat athlete can never achieve his maximum potential.

Many studies show that seeds and nuts are healthy for us, because they make you feel satiated and thus you eat fewer amounts of the unhealthy foods such as burgers, cakes, and pies. This is undeniably a good point, but the truth also is that a handful of nuts is 170–190 calories. Eating one handful a day for a month equals 5,400 extra calories, which corresponds to approximately 1.5 pounds of fat. You need to be aware that nuts are extremely energetically loaded, and you should not be eating more than one or two handfuls a day (unless you are training hard and burning high amounts of energy). Not everybody, myself included, has the self-control needed to stick to one handful of nuts a day. The seeds are easier to control, as they are harder to snack on mindlessly. Keep this in mind, be aware, and stay disciplined with your nuts.

OILS

Now, let us return to the oils. We have all heard how healthy olive oil is in the Mediterranean Diet, haven't we? You may be surprised, but it is not entirely true. While the Mediterranean diet is healthy, it is in spite of the olive oil, and because they eat so many plants. According to Dr. Esselstyn and Dr. McDougall, all oils—saturated (animals), monounsaturated (olive oil), or polyunsaturated (omega-6 and omega-3 oil)—are damaging to the endothelium of the arteries and create new atherosclerotic lesions. Vegetable oils also impair circulation, leading to chest pain, decreased brain function, high blood pressure, reduced lung function, and fatigue. According to Jeff Novick, RD, oils are very nutritionally empty when looking at the amounts of the healthy nutrients per calorie (nutrient density). Therefore, all oils, vegetable or animal, should be eliminated. We want to avoid all processed foods, including the oils. The oils are processed by extraction from the plant. Preferably, eat the plant itself. Avocados, seeds, or nuts will deliver all the fat that you need, plus many other healthy minerals and vitamins that processed oils lack.

Eliminating oils from your menu may be one of the more challenging aspects of your lifestyle change, because we are so accustomed to using oils in everything. We pour olive oil on salads; we add oils in our baking, soups, and other meals. Getting used to a salad without slippery oil may require a slight shift of consciousness. After all, the oil makes the green crunchy leaves slide nicely onto your fork and into your mouth. You have two options: either you learn how to eat your salads non-slippery (I do admit that this was hard at first, because it was difficult to blend the salad) or also you can add some soft beans into it (white beans, butter beans, or cannellini beans). Their consistency is so soft and somewhat slippery, and after blending them into your salad, they partially fall apart and make the green leaves slide just like there is olive oil. Ultimately, make your own dressings from beans, vinegar, and seeds. Once you figure out what you like best, you will never miss oils again.

For many people, transitioning to whole food plant-based nutrition—and without using free (processed) oils—may feel slightly challenging. We are programmed to use oil in almost everything: sautéing, frying, baking, spraying the pan, salads, and many foods. With a little experimentation and an open mind, you will find that preparing foods without oil is equally simple. It is just different, and you will need to change your food preparation habits.

COOKING WITHOUT OIL

Rather than adding oil to your pan, pour one-half to one cup of water, add your vegetables, and cook on medium heat, stirring occasionally until the water evaporates. If the food is still not done, add some more water and keep going. For additional flavors, add soy sauce (Tamari), vegetable broth, red or white wine (alcoholic or nonalcoholic), tomato juice, rice or balsamic vinegar, sherry (alcoholic or nonalcoholic), lemon or lime juice, Worcestershire sauce, salsa, and spices and herbs such as dry mustard, garlic, or ginger root. It will taste great, and you won't miss the oil.

BAKING WITHOUT OIL

The oil in baked goods keeps them soft and moist. Baking without oil may be a little bit more challenging than cooking, but with a little experimenting, you will create some delicious baked goods by replacing the oil with other moist foods such as mashed banana, mashed pumpkin, tofu, applesauce, mashed potato, or tomato sauce. If you occasionally need convenience, there are commercially produced fat replacements on the market.

Your oil-free muffins and cakes may come out a little heavier than goods baked with oils. If you want to have fluffy muffins, use carbonated water instead of tap water. Sometimes, you need to bake your goods a little bit longer. Don't be discouraged when your first creations don't come out just right. With a little trial and error, you will find your ideal oil-free baking routines.

Use parchment paper inside the cake and loaf pans so your baked goods won't stick to the surface of the pan. If they stick anyway, allow them to chill for ten minutes and they will loosen much easier when cool.

[14]

FOODS TO AVOID AND THEIR SUBSTITUTES

Although this list is very short, it may feel emotional and uncomfortable when you read it. You may experience disappointment, anxiety, and even anger that foods are being taken away from you. Remember, you are not forced to do anything. These are only suggestions, and you can ease yourself into them. Decide to be adventurous, take away one group at a time, and see how it goes and how you feel.

To abandon all the unhealthy foods at the same time is an intense experience. It requires dedication, which only a particular type of person can handle. You will need to figure out how to eat without the foods that you are used to, and sometimes a gradual process makes it easier. It really depends on your personality and motivation.

COW OR GOAT MILK, FOR CEREAL, DRINKING OR COOKING

There are many plant-based options out there to use instead of animal milk such as coconut, almond, rice, hemp, or other nut milks. Califia is a national brand that is very tasty. Soy milk is an option too, if used in moderate amounts because of the conflicting research about the benefits or harm. Just stay on the safe side, use it sparingly and always buy organic to make sure that the soy is not genetically modified. The best option is to create a simple and delicious nut or oat milk at home.

For drinking, use plain water, herbal tea, or freshly squeezed juices. Plain water should be your main hydration source. Use juices sparingly because of the added sugar.

BUTTER AND CHEESE

This may be hard for many people as we use butter or cheese in almost every meal. Eventually, you will get used to the natural and clean flavor of your food, but during the transition, you may miss it. It is easy to create your own spread from beans and put it on the bread or in the meals. Different beans will add different flavors. White beans taste and look almost like cheese. During the transition, you can also use the commercially prepared soy or nut cheeses, but I would recommend getting away from them eventually as they are more or less processed. It is simple to create your own delicious nut cheese:

HOMEMADE NUT CHEESE

1. Soak 1 cup of almonds, cashews, walnuts or your favorite nuts overnight in ¾ cup of water.

2. Add three tablespoons of lemon juice, one clove of garlic and a little sea salt and blend everything in a blender until smooth.

3. If you like a strong cheesy flavor, you can add nutritional yeast.

4. Transfer the mass into a nut-milk bag (a reusable filtration bag used for straining fluids) and squeeze out all of the extra liquid.

5. Let it set in the refrigerator overnight.

6. You can eat it now, or if you want a firm cheese, put it in the dehydrator for at least six hours at 115 degrees.

Homemade cheese is simple, quick, and healthy, but dangerously addicting! If your goal is to increase weight, nut cheeses will help you there. If you are, where you want to be, or even get lighter, be aware of the calories and limit the consumption to your needs.

COTTAGE CHEESE, CULTURED MILK, YOGURT, KEFIR, SOUR CREAM

There are some good commercial non-dairy versions of these dairy products. The brand So Delicious is my favorite because they have many products in coconut, almond, or soy variations. You can also create your own yogurt from tofu or nuts, just like the regular milk, and adding a few spoons of lemon juice.

ICE CREAM

Dairy-based ice cream is easy to give up because there are so many delicious non-dairy versions on the market, from coconut, soy, or almond milk. You can also eat pure fruit sorbet or frozen juice bars. It is simple to make your own ice cream by blending frozen fruit of your choice with thick nut milk. The result is yummy, healthy, and nutritious.

MAYONNAISE

If you cannot be without mayonnaise, there are many vegan products, called Vegannaise, to choose from. Making your own vegan mayonnaise at home is very easy.

HOMEMADE VEGAN MAYONNAISE

12-ounce package of firm silken tofu
½ cup soaked (for 4 hours) cashews (drained)
3 tablespoons lemon juice
1 teaspoon mustard
a pinch of sea salt, pepper, or other spices that you like.

Blend all ingredients in the blender until they are smooth.

SOY-FREE VEGAN MAYONNAISE

1 can cannellini beans (drained)
½ large avocado
2 tablespoons apple cider vinegar (or more if you like a stronger flavor)
1 teaspoon maple syrup (or sweetener that you like)
2–3 tablespoons stone-ground mustard
a pinch of salt, and pepper.

Blend everything until smooth.

EGGS

In cooking and baking, you can use Ener-G egg replacer or other brands' egg replacers. In baking, you can substitute eggs with ground flax seeds, tofu, banana, or applesauce. One tablespoon of whole flax seed plus three tablespoons of water substitutes for one egg in recipes.

MEAT, POULTRY, FISH

Along with butter and cheese, giving up eating animal products may be the hardest thing. Our standard western diet is so focused on meat, poultry, and fish and we are indoctrinated from early childhood as to the importance of animal products in the diet. While this belief may be false, it doesn't change your feeling of being cheated when you see a plate without animal products in front of you. Once you overcome the emotional distress and embrace the idea of reducing the pain and death of animals, while improving your health, you will love the concept.

You can fill your plate with all the plants you want and get full before you consume too many calories that would make you fat. Eat starchy vegetables, whole grains, and beans in any combination to your satisfaction. Eat some pasta as well—just use it sparingly, especially if you want to lose weight. Remember, pasta is processed after all.

During the transition period, you may feel like you want to eat something that looks and chews like meat or poultry. If it's hard to get rid of this feeling, add some "meat" products from tofu and soy onto your plate. There are many different brands out there. I recommend cutting down on the "fake meats" eventually, because they are highly processed. As time goes by, and you get used to eating all the different plants, your taste buds adjust, and you won't have any cravings for chewy meat, poultry, or fish. You may even dislike them, though it may be hard to believe right now.

VEGETABLE OILS

Not using any oils for eating or spraying pans can be hard during the transition until you figure out how to do everything.

→ For cooking, use cast iron or stainless steel cookware, and use a tiny amount of water as needed in small quantities to keep food from sticking instead of the oil.

→ For sautéing vegetables, use water, lemon juice, or a little bouillon.

→ For eating, the hardest thing may be a salad that seems too dry without the slippery oil to make it slide down your throat. Try adding cannellini beans into your salad. They will break during blending and become slippery, which will create a pleasing, smooth feeling. You can also make a salad dressing by blending cannellini beans, water, apple cider vinegar, and spices. Orange juice and balsamic vinegar make a nice salad dressing. Nuts can be used with other ingredients in a blender to replace the processed oils.

→ In baking, replace the requested amounts of oil with mashed banana, ground flax seeds, or applesauce. Adding psyllium husk makes your baked goods soft and moist.

Who needs oil after all?

REFINED WHITE RICE AND WHITE FLOUR

Use whole grain (brown) rice, wild rice, or other whole grains. Quinoa is great in sweet or salty dishes. Use whole grain flours; there are many healthy versions out there such as barley, garbanzo, millet, and many more, in a regular or sprouted form.

REFINED AND SUGAR-COATED CEREALS

Pay attention to the labels. Choose whole grain cereals with no added sugars and with very little processing. You can create your own simple cereal by roasting oat flakes (or barley or rye) and adding a few raisins, seeds, nuts, and cinnamon.

CHOCOLATE

Use carob powder or raw cacao in baking. For snacking, find a chocolate bar that is dairy-free, without added oil, and at least 70% of cocoa content. Enjoy only one or two squares to satisfy your craving, but you may find that you won't have any cravings on your new plant-based life style.

COLAS AND SUGAR DRINKS

This is a no-brainer. Sugar-loaded drinks are not suitable for anybody, animal or plant eaters. Drink pure water instead. While this sounds obvious, there are many people out there satisfying their thirst with colas instead of plain water, not understanding how they are destroying their health, gulp by gulp.

COFFEE... WHAT??

Seeing your favorite drink on this forbidden list must feel disappointing. Don't worry, you still can drink your coffee, but I need to bring your attention to it. Excessive drinking of coffee is acid forming in your body. One of the worst coffees is instant coffee. Since we strive for more alkaline and health-promoting environment, we have to be aware of how much coffee we drink.

One or two cups a day are probably fine. Coffee will increase your performance if you drink it before training. If you really care about your health, but still want to drink a lot of coffee, you can experiment with the cold-brewed coffee, Toddy style. It is quick and simple to make, and is less bitter and less acidic, which many people may find more soothing for their stomachs. Soak the ground coffee in cold water for 12 to 24 hours in a refrigerator. Filter before drinking, and enjoy it cold or heated.

This was a very short list of items you should avoid in your new lifestyle. Sometimes the thought of being denied things makes the transition harder. While keeping the list in your mind, imagine how many great new things you can eat instead. Be curious and open minded, and I promise that soon you will love your new lifestyle tremendously.

[15]

THE AMAZING FOODS YOU CAN EAT

When I gradually transitioned into the vegetarian world, I first gave up red meat. I am not good at cooking meat at home, and when I ate out, I just chose something else instead, such as chicken, fish, or tofu. As I was more aware that restaurant eating is hardly ever as healthy as homemade food, I began to eat at home more and went out less, so inherently I was eating less of the poultry and fish. I made exceptions during the holidays so I wouldn't complicate the lives of the host.

As I was cutting down on the animals, poultry, and fish, I occasionally had eggs, but I was crazy about Greek yogurt, kefir, and cheese. I ate them daily and couldn't imagine my life without them. I believed they were necessary for my health. My diet was relatively healthy compared to the general population: I was not eating any fast food, and I was eating a lot of vegetables and fruits. Because I am a person of habit to the extreme, I ate the same vegetables and fruits almost all the time. Perhaps I was not sure how to prepare some of the other more "unknown" (to me) vegetables or was just plain lazy in figuring it out.

Once I gained all the knowledge about animal products and the horrible effects of eating dairy, I made the final decision that I was going to give them up. I had to figure out what I was going to eat. I bought many books, researched many websites, and my eyes began to open wide from excitement—there is a huge, colorful, delicious kingdom of plants. I began to add them, one by one, into my kitchen and experimented with what I can create. I usually ate the plants raw, too. This was amazing.

I began to experience more energy and an indescribable feeling of wellbeing that every plant-based person can confirm. It was so profound that I began to blend fruits and veggies into a smoothie for breakfast before my training. I blended another combination for lunch after the practice, and I cooked several veggie combinations for dinners. I looked into many cuisines of the world and discovered many tasty recipes. I very seldom follow a recipe completely—I see what plants and spices they use and how they put them together. Then I explore what I have in the fridge that could resemble the recipe, and then I put it all together. I have learned that simplicity goes a long way. Especially for busy people and hard training athletes who don't have the luxury of a lot of free time to create complicated meals. The goal is: simple, quick, and delicious. This will guarantee that you will stick to it for life.

Often people wonder what they can eat when they stop eating animal products and dairy. They feel restricted just thinking about it. What you can eat is the smallest problem; the kingdom of plants is so rich that your problem becomes "how do I get all these plants in?" What you can eat is many-fold, compared to what you cannot eat. Note that the lists of the edible plants are far from complete.

FRUITS

Acai
Aceola
Apple
Apricots
Avocado
Banana
Blackberry
Blueberries
Camu Camu berry
Cherries
Coconut
Cranberry
Cucumber
Currants
Dates
Durian

Fig
Goji berries
Gooseberry
Grapefruit
Grapes
Jackfruit
Kiwi
Kumquat
Lemon
Lime
Lucuma
Lychee
Mango
Mangosteen
Melon
Mulberry

Nectarine
Orange
Papaya
Passion Fruit
Peach
Pear
Pineapple
Plum
Pomegranate
Pomelo
Prickly Pear
Prunes
Raspberries
Strawberries
Tangerine/Clementine
Watermelon

A few lesser known, yet very yummy fruits are

Carambola (star fruit)
Cherimoya
Guava

Loquat
Lychee
Pummel

Quince
Soursop/guanabana

VEGETABLES

Artichoke
Arugula
Asian greens
Asparagus
Basil
Beans, green
Beets (all colors)
Bok-Choy
Broccoli
Burdock
Cabbage
Carrots
Cauliflower
Celery
Chicory
Collard greens
Corn
Cucumber

Daikon
Eggplant
Endive
Fennel
Garlic
Horseradish
Hot peppers
Jerusalem artichoke
(sunchoke)
Kale
Kohlrabi
Leeks
Lettuce
Okra
Olive
Onion
Parsley
Peas
Peppers

Pumpkin
Radicchio
Radish
Rhubarb
Salsify
Scallion
Shallot
Spinach
Sprouts (alfalfa, lentil,
mung bean, wheat)
Squash (banana,
butternut, summer,
turban, and other)
Swiss chard
Tomato
Turnips
Water chestnuts
Watercress
Zucchini

STARCHY ROOT VEGETABLES

Jicama
Parsnips
Potatoes

Rutabaga
Sweet potatoes
Tapioca

Taro root
Yams

LEGUMES

Beans:
Adzuki (aduki, azuki)
Black
Fava
Garbanzo (chick-peas)
Great northern
Lima
Mung
Navy
Pink

Pinto
Red kidney
Soy beans
White kidney (cannellini)

Lentils:
Black
Brown
Green
Red

Peas:
Black-eyed
Split green
Split yellow
Whole green

WHOLE GRAINS

Glutenous:
Barley
Einkorn
Emmer
Rye
Triticale
Wheat and its varieties (durum, kamut, spelt, farro, semolina, bulgur, seitan)

Gluten-free:
Amaranth
Buckwheat (or kasha)
Corn
Millet
Oats
Quinoa
Rice (white, brown, wild)
Sorghum
Teff

NUTS AND SEEDS

All can be ground into a nut or seed butter.

Almonds
Brazil nuts
Cashews
Chestnuts
Chia seeds
Coconut

Flax seeds
Hazelnuts
Hemp seeds
Macadamia nuts
Peanuts (theoretically a legume)

Pecans
Pistachio nuts
Pumpkin seeds
Sesame seeds
Sunflower seeds
Walnuts

UNREFINED FLOUR

Barley
Beans
Buckwheat
Corn
Garbanzo

Lima bean
Oat
Potato
Rice

Rye
Soy
Triticale
Wheat

When the whole grain is ground into flour, the physical properties change and the calories from the flour are absorbed faster and completely. If you want to work on losing weight, eliminate flour entirely. Eat sweet or regular potatoes, whole grains, beans, and plenty of vegetables and fruits instead.

EGG-FREE PASTAS AND ORIENTAL NOODLES

Artichoke pasta
Bean threads
Buckwheat soba
Corn pasta
Rice noodles or pasta

Somen
Spinach pasta
Tomato pasta
Udon
Whole wheat pasta

The majority of pastas and noodles are made from highly refined noodles and they should play a very small role in your healthy plant-based diet—just a little treat sometimes.

[16]

SPICES AND SEASONINGS

People who transition to whole foods plant-based nutrition may feel that their meals taste bland at first, because they are not used to preparing plants. Rather than giving up on the plants, adding a few spices and seasonings will make a remarkable difference. If you think about it, you have not been eating unseasoned meat either, have you? Plain meat would be probably rather unappetizing. Plants have many different flavors, smells, colors, and levels of crunchiness, and their combinations create delicious culinary experiences. Most spices are plants in dried, ground, powdered, or liquefied forms, unless they are chemically processed—and we don't eat those.

Grains and legumes without spices can be a little bit boring, but just take a plain chickpea and add a little lemon juice, garlic, and cumin, and you get hummus—a tasty meal from chickpeas.

Don't be shy about using salt during cooking. Salt decreases the bitterness in vegetables and brings all the flavors of your dish together. Bland vegetables taste better as well. Salt helps draw moisture out of sweating vegetables and softens them quicker. Salt also helps to denature proteins (break them apart structurally without losing any nutritional value) for faster digestion and absorption.

Fresh and dried herbs, garlic, ginger, and all other spices add various nutrients to your meals. Grains and beans absorb flavors slowly during cooking, so if you let them marinate in a sauce or dressing with your spices for at least one hour, they will absorb all the flavors and become much tastier. A few ideas on how to add flavor to grains and legumes:

→ Use vegetable broth or juice instead of water for cooking

→ Add spices and herbs to the water while they cook

→ Combine them with fruits or vegetables of your preference

➜ Marinate them in a tangy sauce

➜ Puree them with spices into a dip

➜ Add them to salads or soups

➜ Top them with your favorite pasta sauce

Spices enhance your dishes with vitamins, minerals, proteins, and antioxidants. Use them abundantly and to your liking. Consume a wide variety of spices for great nutritional benefits and exciting flavor combinations. Some spices have a lot of bitterness in them, so start slowly, and increase the amounts over time as you adjust your taste buds, or combine them with plant fats, such as nuts, seeds or avocados. Add whole spices to soups, sauces, and cooking water for grains and legumes, to infuse them with flavor.

Fresh herbs have more nutrition than dried spices, so if you have the opportunity, use them whenever you can. They are rich with vitamins, minerals, and antioxidants. They are great for salads, smoothies, legume dips, and soups. Since fresh herbs wither quickly in heat, you should add them at the end of a hot meal to preserve as much flavor and nutrients as possible. Alternatively, sprinkle them over the completed dish. To release the flavor, rub them between your fingers before adding them to the dish. Experiment with different combinations of spices and plants to find your favorites. As a starter, below you will find a few ideas.

SEASONING COMBINATIONS

Here are some tested, actual flavor combinations that you can start with:

➜ Cinnamon, nutmeg, allspice, ginger, and molasses for oatmeal, porridge, or other cooked grains

➜ Cayenne, cumin, and allspice for a chili with tomatoes, beans, mushrooms, and zucchini

➜ Oregano, basil, and marjoram for tomato sauce or soups

➜ Parsley, thyme, and bay leaves for mushroom gravy, squash risotto, or soups

→ Make your own curry powder from cumin, coriander, ginger, turmeric, and cayenne and use it with chickpeas, sweet potato, and other dishes to give them an Indian flavor

→ Salty soy sauce, tamari sauce, and ginger for broccoli, dark leafy vegetables, and mushrooms

→ Dill, nutritional yeast, garlic, and onion powder for brown rice, cooked grains and steamed vegetables

ANTI-INFLAMMATORY SPICES

The hard-training athlete puts her body through a lot of physiological stress, which causes inflammation that hinders adequate muscle repair. For more rapid recovery, the athlete's goal is to reduce the inflammation as quickly as possible.

TURMERIC

Turmeric and its active ingredient curcumin (which gives the spice its yellow color) is a potent anti-inflammatory and anti-oxidant spice and is worth adding to any food that you make. Turmeric contains 2–5% of curcumin, as well as manganese, iron, vitamin B6, potassium, and fiber. Adding black pepper, which makes it 2000 times more potent, and Mediterranean spices such as thyme, oregano, basil, rosemary, marjoram, and mint doesn't just add colorful flavor, but they can also help to reduce the growth of cancer cells.

Curcumin is a great spice for every serious athlete, improving both recovery and cardiovascular health, as it also decreases the inflammation in the arteries. Combining curcumin with alkaline-forming foods provides additional benefits. Already in 1986, the research showed that a dosage of 1200 mg of curcumin per day was more effective in reducing inflammation than either the placebo or anti-inflammatory medication usually prescribed.

In India, turmeric is considered the standard anti-inflammatory. Indian people use it to keep their tendons and ligaments free from injuries and to minimize pain and inflammation from strenuous activities. Add turmeric to soups, salads, lentils, stews, and other curry dishes. You can also make a curcumin tea, although not very delicious, it is highly potent and healing.

DRIED RED PEPPER

Dried red pepper contains capsaicin, which fights inflammation. Capsaicin makes the dried red pepper flakes spicy. The hotter the peppers are, the more capsaicin they contain and have greater anti-inflammatory benefits. Capsaicin also prevents platelets from clumping together and thus reduces the formation of blood clots. Capsaicin lowers the risk of skin and colon cancers and type-2 diabetes. Its hot taste may decrease your appetite, which is positive if your goal is to lose weight, but if you are highly active, make sure to eat all the calories you need for optimal recovery.

CINNAMON

Cinnamon is anti-inflammatory, antibacterial and anti-clotting, improving cardiovascular health and recovery. Only ¼ or ½ of teaspoon a day added to your oatmeal, smoothies, or juices helps to balance the blood sugar, triglyceride, and cholesterol levels.

GROUND CUMIN

Ground cumin is a potent anti-inflammatory and rich in vitamin C and iron (one teaspoon provides four milligrams). It activates the salivary glands and improves the digestive process. Add it to sautéed vegetables or soups.

NUTMEG

Nutmeg, just like cinnamon, has anti-inflammatory and antibacterial properties. Nutmeg also improves indigestion and insomnia, both beneficial for the hard training athlete. Digesting your foods efficiently will assist the delivery of nutrients to the tissues and a deep sleep is necessary for the recovery. Add some nutmeg powder to your soups, stews, legumes, or sweet potatoes.

GINGER

Ginger contains very potent anti-inflammatory compounds called gingerols, which help to reduce osteoarthritic and rheumatoid pain and swelling, while improving joint mobility. As little as ¼-inch slice of ginger added to your stir-fry, salad dressings, smoothies, or tea is useful, but studies have shown that increased amounts of ginger produce faster and better results. Ginger also provides gastrointestinal relief from nausea, heartburn, or bloating, and improves the immune system.

[17]

SUPPLEMENTS

People often wonder if plant-based diets promote optimal health and performance, and if they are safe and sufficient. The Academy of Nutrition and Dietetics states that well-planned vegan diets are safe and adequate at every stage of the human life cycle, starting with infants, and continuing with children, adults, pregnant or lactating women, athletes, and the elderly. The important notion here is the term "well-planned." One can be a very unhealthy vegan by eating processed vegan foods. That is not a well-planned plant-based diet. A well-planned plant-based diet is safe and adequate, and has some additional benefits of improved athletic performance and decreased risk of chronic diseases.

Almost everybody is taking some sort of supplementation of vitamins and minerals. We have been programmed that popping a pill will cure all the problems we have. We can eat poorly and live an unhealthy lifestyle and the magic vitamin supplements will undo all the damage. Before you take another vitamin supplement, do you know what a vitamin is, actually? The Merriam-Webster medical dictionary defines a vitamin as

> "any of various organic substances that are essential in minute quantities to the nutrition of most animals and some plants, act especially as coenzymes and precursors of coenzymes in the regulation of metabolic processes but do not provide energy or serve as building units, and are present in natural foodstuffs or are sometimes produced within the body."

Notice the two important parts in the definition: present in natural foodstuffs, and in minute quantities.

Every whole food that we eat has many different vitamins, enzymes, and other phytochemicals that work in harmony. Even though we don't need all of them every day, we do need them all. Our bodies have developed over millions of years to proficiently extract all the nutrients from the whole foods we eat. As long as we supply the whole foods, the body will regulate the nutrient intake according to its needs. Supplements are not food. The body doesn't know what to do with the non-food nutrients that usually are in incorrect proportions. The body absorbs nutrients from foods better than from supplements.

The common thought that if something is good then more must be better started the trend of reducing whole foods into new and completely different substances, today known as supplements. We study the food, isolate and test its various substances, and then create a concentrated, chemical version of them. Then we eat the supplements to make up for the lacking nutrients in the modern processed diet. How foolish is this? We first process the foods to take all the nutrients out of it, and later we buy supplements to add the nutrients back in. The problem with this is that the body needs all the thousands of nutrients that act together in interconnected ways that we don't even understand, and taking a few isolated supplements is not going to make up for the missing nutrients that the body would otherwise extract from varieties of whole foods.

There are occasions when using a supplement may be valuable to one's health, for example, when addressing some underlying causes of degenerative conditions. A competent health care professional should always supervise the supplementation. Unfortunately, this is not how supplements are marketed, sold, and used today. They are often marketed as "improve your health" supplements, and in this case, they are not more beneficial than eating whole foods.

On the contrary, they are often harmful to the body because they disturb the natural balance of all the substances in the body. For example, excess vitamin A, E, and beta-carotene increases mortality. You have to treat supplements as medications, not as food. Dr. T. Colin Campbell says that there is no evidence supporting any benefits from consuming isolated nutrients as supplements and that vitamins and minerals should never be consumed in isolation of their naturally occurring state.

By eating a variety of plants and rotating your foods regularly, you will supply your body with everything it needs to extract all the nutrients necessary for optimal health. You don't need any additional supplements other than possibly vitamin B12, calcium, and omega-3 fatty acid (to keep a correct balance with omega-6s). Vitamin D may be another one, but the risk of deficiency is the same in both plant eaters and meat eaters. We just need to make sure to get more of it by exposing ourselves to the sun, safely and with caution. If you have a medical condition, discuss with your medical adviser about your specific case of supplementation.

VITAMIN B12

The vitamin B12 issue in plant-based nutrition is a valid point that we will address. The statement that all plant-based people are deficient in vitamin B12 and thus get horribly sick is a myth that causes fear in many. Some attention needs to be paid to this important vitamin, but we have to keep in perspective the fact that this is only a small "problem" compared to the enormous benefits of plant-based nutrition for our health, reversing chronic diseases, and improving athletic performance. Rather than caused by the diet, vitamin B12 deficiency is usually a symptom of a much larger problem such as digestive disorders, Crohn's or celiac disease, and other gut problems. It manifests as fatigue, weight loss, upset stomach, diarrhea, constipation, numbness, confusion, and memory loss among others.

The requirements of vitamin B12 are very low, but necessary. We need vitamin B12 for cell division and blood formation, but we don't make vitamin B12. Neither do animals or plants.

B12 comes from the coenzymes that are present in bacteria found all around us on Mother Earth. Animals eat the dirt, feces, and bugs and ingest the bacteria that then grow in the animal guts. Therefore, animal products can be a source of vitamin B12. Sometimes, B12 can be found in the soil and on the dirty plants, but we humans don't ingest enough of these microorganisms anymore because we live in a sanitized, cleaned environment.

Even though the recommendation for vitamin B12 is small, you need to add some to your diet occasionally. Vitamin B12 is especially important in pregnancy and lactation and for infants and children. You can add nutritional yeast to your meals to add a cheesy flavor and vitamin B12.

As little as one tablespoon of nutritional yeast will satisfy the recommendations of 2.4 micrograms a day. Nutritional yeast comes in the form of yellow powder and flakes, and is different from brewer's yeast or other yeasts. People sensitive to yeast usually can eat nutritional yeast without problems.

Other sources of vitamin B12 are foods and drinks specially fortified with vitamin B12 such as non-dairy milks, energy bars, cereal, tempeh, and miso. Even though various seaweeds (kombu, wakame, kelp, alaria, dulse, nori) contain high amounts of vitamin B12, the body doesn't seem to absorb it and therefore seaweeds are not acceptable sources of vitamin B12.

Vitamin B12 is a unique vitamin because we need much smaller amounts of it compared to other vitamins, and because it takes at least five years or more to show a deficiency if it happens. The recommendation for B12 intake is 2.4

micrograms a day in the US and around 1–3 micrograms in other countries for the general population. Some studies even suggest raising the levels to 4–7 micrograms per day.

There are many easy methods of getting a sufficient intake of vitamin B12, so you can adopt the one that fits your personality and lifestyle the best. The absorption of vitamin B12 varies dramatically depending how much you are ingesting. If your intake is very low (around one microgram or less), the absorption is very high, about 50%. If your intake is high (around 1000 micrograms or higher), the body absorbs only 0.5%. It means that the less frequently you eat vitamin B12, the greater the total amount needs to be in order to deliver the desired absorbed amount.

VITAMIN B-12 SUPPLEMENTATION

1. If you eat foods fortified with vitamin B12 so that you consume about one microgram of B12 three times a day, it will provide an adequate amount.

2. If you want to eat your vitamin B12 just once a day, then taking a tablet containing ten micrograms would provide an adequate amount of absorbed vitamin B12. For optimal absorption, you should chew the tablet thoroughly and let it dissolve in your mouth completely, or use sublingual forms of vitamin B12.

3. If you are the forgetful type who has a hard time remembering to take supplements, you can make your life simpler by eating one 2,000-microgram tablet just once a week.

No toxicity cases of overdosing on vitamin B12 have been reported; however, you do not need to eat more than 5000 micrograms per week. All three methods are adequate ways to deliver vitamin B12 to your plant-based body if you have a healthy B12 metabolism. However, some individuals may have a compromised absorption of B12, and for them a 2,000-microgram tablet once a week may work the best, because it doesn't rely on a daily required absorption in the gut. If you know or suspect that you have unique metabolic defects, you should contact your medical advisor because you may require other types of administration. These cases are rare, and the majority of us will do fine with the three above-mentioned methods.

Be smart about supplementing with vitamin B12 when you transition to the plant-based nutrition. A vitamin B12 deficiency is hard to notice, because the liver stores B12, which can last for three to six years, and when you start noticing, it could be too late. Give you body regular doses of vitamin B12 and feel great.

CALCIUM

When the plant-based diet is not planned correctly, it may happen that we don't consume enough calcium. We need around 1000 mg per day, but nearly 75% of vegans consume only around 700 mg. About 50% of vegans consume even lower doses, closer to a half of the recommended amount. The calcium intake recommendations for women above 50 years and men above 70 years are 1200 mg, according to research that suggests that adequate calcium and vitamin D intake can reduce the risk of fractures and osteoporosis as people age. Furthermore, exercising regularly will strengthen the bones.

Fortunately, there are high amounts of calcium in plants, yet people are not aware of this fact because they have been incorrectly taught since early childhood that dairy is the only source of calcium. You can get adequate amounts of calcium by eating green leafy vegetables such as kale, turnip greens, broccoli, bok choy, collard, Chinese cabbage, and okra. Collard greens contain as much, if not more, calcium in one cup than one cup of cow's milk.

Some green leafy vegetables, such as spinach, Swiss chard, and beet greens, contain high levels of oxalic acid or oxalates, which jeopardize optimal absorption of the calcium. Make sure you eat a variety of greens and rotating them regularly, in addition to beans, fruits, nuts, and seeds. That way you know that you are consuming and absorbing enough calcium, thus making possible good bone health on your plant-based diet.

There are also high amounts of calcium in tofu. Even though I do not recommend eating tofu in high doses because of the high processing of the soybeans, occasional indulgence is fine.

The amounts of calcium in tofu depend on what coagulating agents have been used in the process; calcium sulfate and magnesium chloride (nigari) are the most common. Tofu made with calcium sulfate usually contains higher amounts of calcium. Analyze the label to calculate the amount of calcium you will get from your tofu. Calcium content is labeled as "percent of daily value", where daily value currently is 1000 mg. Multiply that percent daily value number by ten and you will get how many milligrams of calcium you will get in one serving. For example, tofu with 15% daily value for calcium would have 150 mg of calcium in one serving.

Eat tofu in moderation, as well as all other processed tofu-based products such as TVP (textured vegetable protein), tofu sausages, tofu burgers, and other soy items. Soybeans contain high amounts of enzyme inhibitors that make carbohydrates and proteins from soybeans hard to digest fully. Incompletely digested foods have to be processed by the bacteria in the large intestine, causing discomfort, bloating, or other problems. Fermented versions of soy products, such as miso or tempeh, are a much better choice, because they provide large amounts of friendly microflora in the intestinal tract, which help with digestion and assimilation of nutrients, enhancing immunity.

Stay aware of what you eat and continually educate yourself on the topic of plant-based nutrition and you will thrive in health and athletic performance.

OMEGA-3 AND OMEGA-6 FATTY ACIDS

Fat intake is necessary in every athlete's diet. Fat is calorie dense, with 9 calories per gram, and supplies needed energy for hard training athletes. Fat is essential in many functions of the human body: proper functioning of the cell membranes, insulating and maintaining a healthy temperature, cushioning and protecting vital organs, supplying fatty acids to the brain, and transporting fat-soluble nutrients. Too often, humans consume much higher amounts of fat than needed, and the majority of the fat is the wrong kind that suppresses, rather than supports one's health.

Some fats are very healthy, and two of them are essential to health: linoleic fatty acid (omega-6) and alpha-lineic fatty acid (omega-3). The human body can synthesize many of the needed fats from the whole foods that you eat, but not the omega-6 and omega-3 fatty acids. They are essential for normal functioning of all tissues, for the formation of healthy cell membranes, and the proper development and functioning of the brain and nervous system. Many of their positive health benefits are reduced risk of heart disease and stroke, prevention of atherosclerosis, and reduced pain and inflammation.

We need both omega-6 and omega-3 fatty acids for optimal health. These two essential fatty acids compete for the same enzymes that break down the fat molecules into acids during de-saturation. Eating too much of one of them causes too little of the other one and leads to health problems and disease.

Many sources suggest that the optimal ratio of omega-6s to omega-3s is approximately 2:1 or 1:1. The standard Western diet is excessive in omega-6s and deficient in omega-3s with the ratios 15:1 up to 50:1. These high ratios promote disease to an extreme, including heart disease, cancer, and inflammatory and autoimmune diseases. Eating whole foods plant-based nutrition will reduce the ratios of omega-6s to omega-3s to nearly perfect levels because the plant diet is lower in omega-6s than a standard processed food diet. The majority of fats in the whole food plant-based diet are predominantly omega-3s. Generally, no additional supplementation is necessary, but you need to continue paying attention and continuously include good sources of omega-3s and omega-6s daily.

OMEGA-6 FATTY ACIDS

Omega-6 fatty acids are found in legumes, grains, nuts, and seeds. Vegetable oils, such as safflower, sunflower, sesame, soybean, cottonseed, and corn, contain high amounts of omega-6 fatty acids. Many health unconscious vegans falsely believe that they are doing good things for their health by consuming all these vegetable oils, and unknowingly reach ratios of omega-6 to omega-3 as high as 120:1. A smart whole food plant-based athlete should avoid all these oils entirely.

OMEGA-3 FATTY ACIDS

Omega-3 fatty acids should be taken on a daily basis. Foods rich in omega-3s are green leafy vegetables (56%), fruits, beans, nuts, and seeds. One of the best sources of omega-3s is flaxseeds and flaxseed oil (53–62%), chia seeds (57%), and hemp seeds (20%). Other oils, such as canola (11%), walnut (10%), wheat germ (7%), and soybean (7%) also contain omega-3s, but the whole food sources are more desirable.

One tablespoon of ground flaxseeds or one teaspoon of flaxseed oil will supply the daily requirement of alpha-linolenic acid (ALA, one of the omega-3s), which is 1.6 grams for men and 1.1 grams for women. Additionally, flaxseeds are an exceptional source of lignans, a potent anti-carcinogen.

Be aware that flaxseeds are susceptible to rapid damage through oxygenation, heat, and light, and they turn rancid quickly. You should store them in the refrigerator or freezer in an airtight and opaque container and grind the desired amount just before eating them, using a high-powered blender or coffee grinder for a few seconds.

Add the ground flaxseeds in your smoothie, salad, breakfast, or any dish. While it is possible to over consume omega-3 fatty acids (over 3,000 milligrams a day), it is not that common. If you eat a whole foods diet, you do not face that risk. Thanks to persistent marketing of supplements, most people believe that fish oil contains the highest quality omega-3 fatty acids, The truth is that fish omega-3 molecules are extremely unstable. They disintegrate rapidly, releasing dangerous free radicals in the process. Omega-3s found in vegetables, fruits, beans, and seeds are much more stable than fish oil.

Mahatma Gandhi expressed it correctly:

*"Whereever flaxseeds become
a regular food item among the people,
there will be better health."*

TAURINE

While it is not talked about much for the general population, taurine is an amino acid that may improve performance in athletes, and especially plant-based athletes who may be low in taurine in special cases. Animal products are primary sources of taurine, and the plant-based athlete needs to be aware of his or her nutritional choices. Lack of taurine in plant-based athletes can make them anxious. Combined with added stress from training, this can be an unfavorable situation for the hard training athlete.

Taurine lowers the cortisol levels and thus helps to decrease stress and anxiety. Additionally, it supports insulin health, lowers blood pressure, protects the heart, helps with detoxification, elevates energy production, helps to fight inflammation, and improves the reaction times of athletes. Taurine appears to be a great supplement for improved performance. For maximum benefit, make sure that your omega-3 to omega-6 ratios are balanced, as described in the previous chapter.

Taurine is synthesized in the pancreas if there are sufficient amounts of the amino acid cysteine, in combination with methionine, pyrodixine (vitamin B6) and vitamin C. Plant-based sources of cysteine are broccoli, Brussels sprouts, garlic, granola, oats, onions, red peppers, and wheat germ. High levels of methionine are found in Brazil nuts, sesame seeds, seaweed, and spirulina. Broccoli, cooked corn, potatoes, turnip greens, and spinach contain significant amounts of methionine as well. Vitamin B6 is also found in vegetables, nuts, and whole grains.

All of these sources are part of the daily plant-based menu, and so taurine deficits should not be a problem unless you train hard and don't eat an adequate amount of calories and nutrients (especially cysteine, methionine, or B6), or if you are deficient in the enzyme needed to make taurine (can be found in brewer's yeast). If you have candida, you lose taurine through urine.

Taurine is stored in the bile of the gallbladder and helps the body metabolize fat, making it essential for energy production and a lean physique. Hard training athletes often deplete taurine levels during energy production. Taurine is also concentrated in the skeletal muscle tissue, and with muscle damage, taurine is excreted in the urine.

If you are an athlete with low taurine levels, a safe supplementation dosage is one gram per day. To improve brain function, two to three grams a day are recommended. To efficiently protect heart function, up to six grams a day may be taken. There is no evidence of negative health effects from taurine supplementation.

In athletes with low levels of muscle taurine, an effective supplementation will increase force production, improve both aerobic and anaerobic endurance, speed up the recovery from intense training, and increase the workload capacity.

[18]

ORGANIC OR CONVENTIONAL

As stated earlier, organic is like a private school for food. If you can afford it and find it close to you, choose it. If it is difficult to find organic produce, eating conventional produce has more health benefits than not eating it at all. Don't let the lack of access to organic foods prevent you from reaching your potential in health, sports, and life.

Dr. Bruce Ames of the University of Berkley has devoted his entire career to studying the residual pesticides on the foods and their effects on human health. He and his research team believe that humans ingest thousands of various toxic substances that are naturally present in fruits and vegetables, and their bodies have higher toxic levels than the residual toxins on the foods.

Other scientists believe that there is a chance that some chemicals increase toxicity. In a study that reviewed data gathered by the U.S. Department of Agriculture, researchers compared 8 fruits and 12 vegetables and found that 73% of the non-organic crops contained pesticide residues, in comparison to 6–27% of organic crops. For some non-organic fruits (apples, peaches, pears, and strawberries) and for one non-organic vegetable (celery), over 90% of the non-organic food samples showed pesticide residues. The toxicity topic is still studied without any absolute conclusions.

Independent of the contrasting views, the scientists all agree on one thing: you should never reduce or completely stop eating vegetables and fruits just because they may contain toxins. All cancer research to this date shows that the higher the amounts of fruits and vegetables we eat, the lower our risk of cancer and heart disease. All the studies used conventionally grown produce, and clearly showed that the benefits outweigh the potential risks. However, if it is under your control, you should try to reduce the exposure to toxins as much as you can.

Avoid the skins of the fruits that have the highest pesticide residue. Always wash your produce before eating. According to the Environmental Group's "Shopper's Guide to Pesticides" you should avoid conventionally grown "dirty dozen" foods that consistently show the highest pesticide values. The list is rated from the highest contaminated to the least contaminated and you should always choose an organically grown version:

1. Celery	**5.** Blueberries	**9.** Cherries
2. Peaches	**6.** Nectarines	**10.** Kale
3. Strawberries	**7.** Bell peppers	**11.** Potatoes
4. Apples	**8.** Spinach	**12.** Imported grapes

The least contaminated fruits are pineapples, mangoes, kiwifruit, papayas, watermelon, grapefruit, and avocado. Even then, you should wash them well and peel the skin.

The least contaminated vegetables are onions, broccoli, cabbage, sweet corn, asparagus, sweet peas, eggplant, tomatoes, and sweet potatoes. Wash your veggies carefully with the special produce wash because plain water removes only 25–50% of the pesticides. Discard the outer leaves of conventional cabbage and lettuce.

[19]

PLANT-BASED RESTAURANT EATING

The number of restaurants with plant-based foods is increasing, in some areas more, and in others, they are just catching up. The rising problem is the quality of vegan restaurant foods. Even though a vegan meal will assure you that the meal is free of any animal products, there is no guarantee about the quality of the meal. The meal can contain high amounts of fat, saturated fat, added oils, sugars, salt, processed grains that lack nutrients and fiber, and other additives. This is still junk food—animal-free junk food.

It is difficult to find good options for your plant-based life style when you have to travel. People are seldom aware that vegan restaurants can be this bad for you. They believe that as long as they eat "vegan" they are doing good things for their health. Many times, the restaurants promoting vegan, vegetarian, and raw options are surprisingly unhealthy, in addition to being very expensive. For example, vegan lasagna consists of processed vegan cheese, a lot of added oils, and contains few vegetables. This is not a healthy meal.

I used to be a fan of the Veggie Grill that serves great tasting vegan burgers and traditional meals cooked with no animal products until I looked at the nutrition labels. To my surprise, the amounts of fat were in the range of 20–30 grams per meal, which is almost the recommended allowance for the entire day. No wonder the place is always crowded: people love the taste of fat, and they are fooled into thinking that the food is healthy because it is vegan. One can argue that it is better to eat a fatty vegan burger rather than a fatty meat burger and in a way, it is true, because at least we are saving the lives of innocent animals. However, when considering food as the means to health, longevity, and athletic performance, then the fat-laden vegan burger is not good.

If you travel and need to dine in restaurants, you almost have a better chance of finding a good plant-based meal in a "regular" restaurant or a steak house. You can skip the chicken or steak part of the meal and order a baked potato or sweet potato with steamed vegetables and green salad.

You will find great choices in ethnic restaurants: in Asian restaurants choose brown rice, steamed edamame without salt and steamed vegetables; in the Mexican places, choose beans and rice and steamed vegetables; in Indian restaurants you find lentils, rice, steamed vegetables; in other restaurants you may find various grains, steamed and lightly prepared in addition to rice and vegetables.

Other national chain restaurants where you can find vegan meals are Chipotle Mexican Grill, California Pizza Chicken, Souplantation/Sweet Tomatoes, Panera Bread, P.F. Chang's, Chili's and many more.

One simple rule to remember: eat a variety of unrefined and minimally processed foods that are naturally rich in fiber and nutrients. Often you can build your own menu from the side dishes, or order a main dish without the animal part. Design your own meal that is low in fat, saturated fat, omega-6 fatty acids, cholesterol, added sugars, added salt, added oil, and refined grains. It may seem very restrictive at first glance, but there is an array of possibilities and diversities in the plant world and the restaurants and kitchens tend to be very helpful if you politely ask them.

Switching to a plant-based diet feels tricky at first because it looks more complicated than it is. If you are motivated enough and keep learning and educating yourself, you will get it down in no time.

SECTION 3

EFFECTS OF NUTRITION ON THE BODY

[20]

MODERATION

When people encounter the idea of whole foods plant-based nutrition for the first time, they usually think it is rather extreme. They defend their indoctrinated eating habits with the words "everything in moderation" and claim that moderation in foods and exercise is the best. While this could be theoretically true, in reality it is far from that. There are some people who do well on moderation, but for the majority of people, moderation doesn't work.

For an athlete, moderation in exercise is usually impossible. Athletes generally exercise too much, which is the side effect of what they chose to become—a high performing individual. Every competitive athlete is pushing his or her physical limits to an extreme, as do many of the recreational athletes and fitness warriors as well. The elite athlete's livelihood depends on their extreme fitness levels, and many recreational athletes compete in local competitions where maximum performance becomes their goal and driving motivation. Therefore, they will not exercise in moderation. Because of that, it is crucial to implement strict nutritional practices. Athletes need to repair their challenged bodies for performance and longevity. Moderation won't do it.

There is another problem with moderation. Say you allow yourself to eat some of the bad stuff, but not too much. A little cheese, chocolate, or fatty meal should be ok, right?

But how do we define "too much" and when is enough enough? How do we know if we have surpassed the limit? This is a serious problem: we don't know! We all have different taste buds and levels of registering the pleasure from eating. For example, if you eat sweet foods often, your taste buds down-regulate and you don't taste the sweetness as much as the person who seldom eats sweets. For the other person, one cookie would be too much, but for your taste buds, three or five cookies may not do it. The same goes for all flavors, drugs, and other indulgent behaviors.

Moderation is challenging for many people. Once they have a small amount of addictive food (for them), it will cause so-called priming, which is a similar response to food that alcoholics have to the taste of alcohol. While we don't completely understand the priming's mechanism in the brain, we know that a small amount of certain foods for some people will create a strong, often uncontrollable drive to eat more. Different people have different addictive foods; some have chips or crackers, others sweets and cakes, or others fats and heavy foods. These foods produce certain emotions and create strong and everlasting addictions when people take pleasure in these emotions too much. A tiny piece of the food makes you want to have more. This is the reason that moderation is impossible and why we have so many overweight people around. They mean well with moderation, but they don't have any control over it. That is why people fight so strongly for their foods when they hear they need to give them up. The addict inside, consciously or subconsciously, is fighting.

Americans consume, on average, two and a half times more added sugar than recommended, twice as much refined grains and sodium than recommended, and three times more fats than recommended. Even if they choose to consume these foods in moderation, it won't be good enough because they are so high above the recommended threshold already. They need to reduce consumption of added sugars, refined grains, added fats, and sodium by at least half just to reach the upper level of recommended servings.

Looking at the opposite end—the good foods, such as vegetables, fruits, and grains—Americans eat, on average, only half of the recommended minimum intake of fruits, vegetables, and fiber, and only 15% of whole grains. Even in this case, moderation is not acceptable, because just to reach the bare minimum, a dramatic increase is needed: twice as much of the fruit, vegetables, and fiber, and seven times more whole grains. One third of Americans are obese, two thirds are overweight, and 70% of Americans don't meet the minimum recommendations for exercise. I believe that these numbers do not represent the readers of this book, but it is still something to ponder.

Athletes are more extreme people, and they need more extreme measures. They are much more active, and they need to eat much better than the average person to achieve optimal recovery and peak potential. Moderation in nutrition for athletes will bring moderate results. Everybody who succeeds in something is mildly obsessive, and this is true about nutrition as well. Dr. Esselstyn's memorable saying to his cardiac patients is "moderation kills." For the high performance athlete, moderation slows you down. If you want extreme results, take extreme measures.

[21]

LOSING WEIGHT

Many people struggle with their weight and they try different diets all through their lives. A few diets work to some degree for a short time, but 95% of dieters regain all their weight and more within one to three years. Losing weight and becoming lean is not a matter of a few months' quick fix, even though it is possible to do, but rather it is a lifetime change of lifestyle. If you want to become lean, fit, and healthy and remain that way forever, you will need to look into how you eat.

While people want to look lean and athletic, the looks on the outside don't necessarily correlate to the health on the inside. The main priority of every person and athlete should be improving their health first, through good nutrition. As a bonus, you will also lose weight, feel more energy, look more radiant, and perform better. The lifestyle change when focusing mainly on your health rather than your looks will also increase motivation, vitality, mental clarity, and enthusiasm for life.

Sometimes people choose to become vegetarians or vegans just to lose weight. Yet, I have seen so many unhealthy or overweight vegetarians and vegans. Avoiding meat, poultry, and dairy isn't a sure path to weight loss if you eat other high-calorie foods excessively, such as nuts, processed pasta, vegetarian fatty cheeses, and oily non-meaty foods. Becoming a vegan is a good step, but you have to be aware that it is not an automatic process, even though it usually happens.

As mentioned before, think about your new lifestyle and decide the best reasons for you. It should be your health first, because when you lose your health, you have nothing worthwhile left. Medical treatments usually deal only with the symptoms of some underlying and more serious issue that presented itself in the form of a disease. You are the only one who can take care of yourself, even better than any medical practitioner. While you may need medical attention sometimes, at the deeper level, your health is in your hands and nutrition is your tool for success.

As an athlete, you may choose new nutritional practices to improve your performance, and you will be very pleased to notice that your health will improve as well. They go hand in hand. If your body's immune system functions well, you will recover faster; you can train harder and with abundant energy; you will perform at higher intensities.

As we age, our metabolism slows down, and we accumulate a little bit of extra weight. Usually we think it is a part of aging, but I don't believe so. Just because this is happening to the average person, it doesn't mean that we have to be average. You can remain fit at any age, but you do have to work on it with discipline. The beauty of whole foods plant-based nutrition is that your body gets all the essential nutrients in abundance and without any toxic substances that slow down your metabolism. You will notice that you feel and look better despite your chronological age.

I always have to remind my mom, who is approaching her 70s—and I need to say I truly respect her efforts and fitness level at her age—that just because it is "normal" that every person that is over sixty years old has high blood pressure and other ailments, it doesn't need to be "normal" for her. The "normal" in our modern society is the average of all people, but if they don't take care of themselves and become fatter and sicker, then the average is sicker too. We don't want to be like the average person. It is not necessary to be overweight and unhealthy, at any age. We all can be better than the average.

LOSING WEIGHT TOO FAST

There are people, and you may have encountered them, who say they really tried to be plant-based or vegan, but it didn't work for them because they got sick and thus had to go back to eating animal products. Most of the time, people who don't thrive on plant-based nutrition don't eat enough calories and as a result they lack energy, feel dizzy or weak, or just simply don't feel right. We are conditioned to believe, falsely, that carbohydrates are bad for us, including even the health-promoting carbohydrates such as potatoes, rice, corn, and fruits.

When people start eating plants, they consciously (or unconsciously, from fear) avoid the complex carbohydrates and they don't consume enough calories. When all the fatty animal products are gone from the menu, we have to eat more calories from plants. With the low energy density, plants will provide a lot of volume, but people tend to continue eating the same amounts as they used to when they were eating animal products. They start losing weight quickly, which they love in the beginning, but this eventually backfires and they become tired and lethargic. They blame the plants.

Depending on your metabolism and activity levels, you need to deliver all the calories needed for optimal performance and wellbeing. If you love to eat, the plant-based approach is excellent for you because the volumes of food you can eat are amazing and without adding too many calories. Don't rush the weight loss… it will occur as a side effect of your newly adopted lifestyle. If you are losing weight too fast, and you don't feel energetic, or your performance suffers, eat more of the calorie-dense plants such as potatoes, rice, grains, seeds, nuts, and dried fruits. If you are losing too slowly or not at all, eliminate the calorie densest foods first and adjust accordingly.

Once you reach your weight goal, add them slowly back in amounts that will not cause unwanted weight gain. As you get lighter, healthier, and fitter, your metabolism increases and you will be able to eat more. Pay attention to how you feel, how you perform, and mental state, and try to maintain a good balance by increasing or decreasing your calorie intake accordingly. Regardless of the calorie levels, always strive for variation and eat from the entire spectrum of the plant world.

[22]

GAINING WEIGHT

While the majority of people seem to want to lose weight, there are athletes, who struggle to gain weight. Unless you are in this category of "hard gainers", it may be difficult to understand how challenging it can be to gain a few pounds of muscle mass. To gain one to two pounds per week, you need to eat extra 500–1000 calories per day, which can total 2,500–3,500 calories per day and even more for athletes. By volume, that is a lot of food. Unless you love to eat and chew, you may have difficulties consuming such volumes of clean, healthy whole foods.

An easy way to increase the calories is by including more nuts, seeds, and nut butters into your diet.

Also, make sure to eat sufficient amounts of carbohydrate dense foods (foods that contain many carbohydrates per serving), because they help you replenish your muscle glycogen stores so you can train with greater intensity and for longer periods. The ingested plentiful carbohydrates will preserve the protein for building -muscle mass rather than burning it for energy to cover insufficient energy intake. Some of the most carbohydrate dense foods are cassavas, taro roots, plantains, yams, potatoes, raisins, dates, persimmons, bananas, and mangos.

A person needs about 0.8 grams of protein per kilogram of body weight (0.36 g/lb) and if you want to gain weight, then you need about 0.9 grams (0.4 g/lb). For athletes, the numbers are 1–1.5 g/kg (0.46–0.68 g/lb), depending how hard they train. Eating plant-based whole foods should deliver the correct amounts of protein, but if the athlete has difficulties eating enough calories, then further supplementation of plant-based protein may be necessary. A moderately active 160-pound person who wants to gain weight should eat an extra 73 grams of protein per day and a hard-training athlete should eat an extra 109 grams per day. This is easily achievable if you eat a high calorie diet, but for people not used to eating a lot, the amounts of food are hard to imagine, and swallow. Often people who struggle with gaining weight don't eat enough.

These are simple guidelines for the daily amounts of food: ten to twelve or more servings of grains, four to eight servings of legumes, four or more servings of fruits, four or more servings of vegetables, four or more servings of healthy fats. For people who love to eat, this is a heaven of deliciousness.

Pay attention to your current nutritional program and how many calories you eat. If you are not meeting your caloric needs, add nuts, seeds, avocados, nut milks, and other denser foods into your menu. Baked vegan goods are a delicious addition of compact calories. Add nuts and seeds to your smoothies, oatmeal, salads, baked goods, and as snacks to carry around. Add avocados to your smoothies, soups, salads, and dips. Create your own nut milks that you use with your cereals, for cooking, baking, and drinking. Create your own homemade baked goods with nuts, dried fruits, seeds, and nut butters. They are healthy and nutritionally dense. Using a high-powered blender, you can create raw versions of nut and fruits bars that are quick to make, delicious, and nutritious.

Eat more often, at least five to six times per day. Eat before you go to sleep and don't go too hungry for too long. Eating an extra 500 calories every day will result in about one pound of weight gain per week. Stay focused on your goal. Make sure that you drink between meals rather than with meals because the fluids that you drink during your meals will fill you up so you won't be able to eat as much, and also they will dilute the digestive juices in your stomach and compromise the digestion of food. If you really struggle with adding on extra pounds, drink fruit juices or nut milks instead of plain water, which will increase the calories in your diet effortlessly.

Make sure that you have food accessible anywhere, anytime: in your car, at your office, in your sport bag, and all other places where you spend time. Always have some nuts, dried fruit, homemade baked goods, or energy bars handy. Pay attention to how your body feels when you eat these large amounts of food. Some people feel that their digestion works better in the morning hours, for others it is in the late hours. Adjust accordingly and consume the heavier meals during the times of your optimal digestion. You can possibly add digestive enzymes to your meals during the hours when your digestive power is not optimal. Healthy eating is a life-long experiment between you and your food. Observe and adjust accordingly.

[23]

PHYTOCHEMICALS AND ANTI-NUTRIENTS

There is a slight paradox regarding the health benefits of eating plants. The experts who promote eating animal products especially love this paradox and use it to prove their point.

Since plants cannot run away from predators, they need to protect themselves in a different way. Most legume seeds contain phytates—compounds that effectively prevent or slow down the absorption of vitamins, minerals, and other nutrients from the intestinal tract of animals that eat them. Therefore, phytates are sometimes labeled as anti-nutrients. The more the animal eats, the less nourishment it gets and starts losing weight. The animals will learn quickly what foods are good or bad for them. For humans, cooking or sprouting the beans and grains will lessen the phytates' effect, even though it won't completely eliminate them. This is not as big a problem as the anti-grain experts tend to present to scare people from adopting a plant-based diet.

Another anti-nutrient is a compound that mimics essential proteins and enzymes necessary for cell division and growth. When the insect eats the nutrient, it enters the cells, preventing their division and growth, and the insect eventually dies. In modern medicine, cancer specialists use this great idea to slow down or stop rapid division of cancer cells.

We don't need to worry about dying from eating plants though. Humans have cohabited and developed with plants for millions of years and learned to eat these compounds, which act like micro doses of chemotherapy—they stop and destroy the fast-dividing cancer cells that always flow around the body. Eating many plants creates a low-level toxicity that activates the longevity genes. Eating plants is like getting micro vaccines that prevent future diseases.

Phytochemicals often demonstrate completely different properties than standard nutrients such as vitamins, minerals, and amino acids. Millions of phytochemicals found in common foods have healing properties that we still don't know about. Currently, this subject is being studied extensively. Eating a variety of plants will deliver a perfect mixture of nutrients and phytochemicals for optimal health.

[24]

HORMESIS AND DETOX

Natural health practitioners use the term "detoxing symptoms" that consist of headaches, fevers, chills, skin rashes, lethargy, nausea, dizziness, and other unpleasant conditions. This usually happens when you switch from the unhealthy Western eating habits to healthy whole foods plant-based nutrition, raw foods, or juicing. The explanation is that the body is releasing all the accumulated toxins stored in the fat cells. The symptoms will pass, and you will feel revitalized and energized.

However, another theory is that these symptoms are the result of a rapid large exposure to plant toxins that the body is not accustomed to, and the liver enzymes cannot process them fast enough. The detox diet is essentially a toxin diet. Nevertheless, toxins in this case are good. Dr. Stephen Gundry treated many overweight patients with bypass surgery, after which the patients lost 100–150 pounds rapidly, and they did not show any signs of detox symptoms, even though their body was releasing huge amounts of heavy metal toxins from their shrinking fat cells. Being lightly poisoned by the plants is similar to feeling sick after getting a vaccine.

HORMESIS

Hormesis is a biological phenomenon where the body has a positive response, such as improved health, stress tolerance, growth, or longevity, which results from exposure to low doses of a substance that is otherwise toxic or even lethal when taken at higher doses. It's sort of like the Nietzche's quote: "That which does not kill you, makes you stronger." When you manage this biological phenomenon wisely and methodically, you will achieve great health benefits of improved health, strength, resilience, and longevity.

Hormesis refers to the beneficial effects of something that would otherwise be harmful at higher levels. It improves resistance to infection, disease, cancer tumors, and aging. It strengthens the immune system, which allows you to train harder and recover better. Researchers at the University of Wyoming found surprising results where mice subjected to low doses of radiation through their lives lived on average 30 percent longer that their siblings without radiation. The radiation didn't kill them, it made them stronger, just like Nietzsche said. Similar studies with other environmental stressors such as lack of nutrients, cold, heat, or ultraviolet light resulted in the same conclusions: all the stressors in low doses promoted survival rather than killing the subjects.

Another example of hormesis is calorie restriction. Studies show that limiting calorie intake improves health and increases longevity. There is an important distinction, however: eating fewer calories while getting all the nutrients from the whole foods will extend the life span; eating empty calories from junk foods and just eating smaller amounts of them will not. Even though the levels of cortisol and adrenaline rise slightly during calorie restriction, they act as hormetic stressors. According to Dr. Steven Grundy, "the hormetic stressors activate genetic programming and stimulate metabolic pathways to resist the environmental challenges and to increase the chances of survival during hostile conditions by increasing healthy life span, rejuvenation, and regeneration." Many studies on longevity suggest that if you eat fewer calories, you will live longer.

Similar reactions occur during exercise and training. Exercise is a stressor that makes the body adapt so it can resist similar stressors in the future and your athletic performance improves over time. The stressors or toxins produce a response that makes your body not just endure the stressor, but improve and thrive. Countless studies suggest that moderate exercise (as a hormetic stressor) increases lifespan while too much exercise may reduce your lifespan. Small doses of exercise improve your immune system as a response to the hormetic stressor. However, when the stress is too high, your immune system becomes compromised. This is a tricky dance along the edge for every competitive athlete. When is too much too much?

Every athlete has a difficult decision to make. When you exercise, you need to eat more calories. How does the increased demand for calories needed for higher doses of exercise correlate to longevity? The mice on a restricted calorie intake looked exactly the same as the mice eating more and exercising. However, the lower-calorie mice lived longer than the fitness mice. This is not very good news for athletes and passionate fitness enthusiasts. When you exercise more, you need to eat more, but you may be risking your longevity. There are other important points to consider. When you exercise, you feel energized and happy, and your immune system becomes stronger, thus preventing possible disease that could reduce your lifespan. You most probably don't carry excess fat weight or suffer with metabolic diseases caused by being overweight, which prolongs your lifespan. Several other factors can affect your health and longevity, and after a thorough consideration, you will need to figure out your own plan and goals. One thing is sure: eating whole foods plant-based nutrition is one good way to excellent health and performance.

HORMESIS AND PLANTS

Many plants contain toxins, which can be disabled by special enzymes during germination when sprouting. For example, beans are quite toxic, while their sprouts are non-toxic and can be safely eaten. Small amounts of toxins, conforming to hormesis, are great for your health. It is always better to eat many different plants in smaller amounts than one plant in large quantity.

All vegetables have hormetic characteristics, but bitter vegetables seem to be much stronger. To use hormesis to your health advantage, make sure that you eat many vegetables and leafy greens in their raw form. Start slowly so you won't experience a too-strong toxic response with headaches, rashes, diarrhea, or joint pain. Initially, you can cook the majority of your plants, but gradually exchange some of them for raw. Increase the raw amount as you get used to them and your immune system becomes stronger. Cook your vegetables for a shorter time than you would usually. They will be half-cooked-half-raw, kind of yummy, firm, and crunchy. Eventually, you will get used to the texture of the parboiled (partially cooked) vegetables and never want to eat the fully cooked ones again. You can also quickly stir-fry them in a tiny amount of water or lemon juice.

[25]

CRAVINGS AND MICROBES

Almost everybody has tried some kind of diet in his or her lifespan. Various diets were popular during different time periods, and we have all tried at least a few. Some extreme cases, usually women, go from diet to diet, like milestones on their life journey. There is always a "valid" reason: we need to fit special clothes for a special occasion, we need to drop weight really fast to look good for the summer, or we are just not happy with how life goes and we believe that losing weight will make it go better. And even though we are aware that there are no shortcuts, every new diet that pops up on the market still gives us false hope. Whether the diet is somehow sound or completely messed up, we all know about the extreme cravings during these diets.

CRAVINGS

Even if you are not on any particular diet, you probably feel cravings sometimes as well—the annoying, irresistible temptations that lure you into eating something you should not eat. You feel great while eating it, and you feel bad immediately afterwards because you feel guilty. The nature of cravings is both physiological and emotional. Some foods trigger certain centers in the brain just as a drug addiction would. From early childhood, we have learned to associate certain feelings with certain foods, and when we feed the emotions with these foods, strong bonds, are created and reinforced, and are hard to break. With these foods, no amount of willpower will help. You can resist for some time, but eventually the craving will overpower you. This usually happens when you have tough moments emotionally. Each time you succumb, you make this addiction stronger.

When I tell people about my whole foods plant-based nutrition, they respond with

"I cannot imagine life without meat."

"I love cheese so much."

"I can't give up milk."

"What would my life be without ice cream?"

While I do have several good answers, such as there are delicious ice creams based on coconut or soy milk, there are nut versions of milk, or tofu based versions of meat and poultry, the question really is why they think they cannot live without these products? Do they need them to feed their body, or do they need them to feed their emotions and psyche?

We all should have a little introspection on why we eat certain foods, especially the ones without which we cannot imagine to be in this world. What is the motivation behind eating these foods? What are we coping with, hiding behind, or escaping from? All these reflections are food for thought (pun intended) that can be difficult but extremely useful not just for your eating habits but also for your life practices in general. When you discover your deep thoughts, motivations, fears, pains, and inner drives, you will act much calmer in stressful situations, because you will be aware of how you tend to react. Processing these thoughts will give you more control of your diet and life, because you will be able to choose what is best for you and your body rather than reacting to emotions with automatic cravings. Once you understand yourself emotionally, the transition will be much easier.

MICROBES' ROLE IN CRAVINGS

Another insight that makes your dietary change easier is the understanding of the physical level of your food preferences and addictions. These are called microbes. Our gut flora contains about forty thousand different bacterial strains. Our entire body is a host of trillions of microorganisms, such as bacteria, fungi, and many other invisible "residents" that symbiotically occupy our organs, skin, saliva, and digestive tract. While our body is comprised of about ten trillion cells, these microorganisms are many times more. Theoretically, we are one big microbe. These microbes are our friends that break down foods that we cannot digest. To achieve optimal health and performance we need to have a healthy microbial system ecology.

Many researchers have been looking at the microbes and connection to food cravings, and the results are astonishing, confirming microbial cravings. This is great news for you, because if you can change your microbes, you can change your cravings. The Swiss scientists performed a small study and determined that people who crave daily chocolate have different microbe colonies in their digestive system than people who are not enticed by chocolate's seductiveness. The study took a long time to complete because it was extremely difficult to find individuals who don't care for chocolate. Researchers suggest that this might be the case for other foods as well. By changing the composition of the trillions of bacteria in your intestines and stomach, you can change the cravings for foods. Dr. Sam Klein, an obesity expert and professor of medicine at Washington University in St. Louis, said that intestinal bacteria change when people lose weight. This is becoming a hot field of scientific research. Certain scientists believe that there is a link between our intestinal microbial ecology and our way of thinking.

If you personally battle with certain food addictions, this is great news for you. Rather than fighting your cravings, be proactive and break the cycle by replacing all the unhealthy foods that you crave with healthy plant-based foods, which will produce completely different microbial flora in your digestive system. Once you create your new healthy colony, these microbes will send signals to your brain with powerful cravings for healthy and nourishing foods. You may not believe this now, but very soon you will be craving a nice green kale and banana smoothie instead of ice cream, or a sprouted grain and lentil loaf instead of a hamburger. To your satisfaction, you will find that the pesky cravings that used to occupy your mind and undermine your self-control are all gone. Eating and becoming healthy is truly easy now.

TASTE IS ACQUIRED

Some people may argue that it is hard to be proactive and build a new happy family of good microbes by changing what we eat, because they don't like the taste of the healthy foods, and it is hard to eat them. It is a valid point with a simple solution. The average person has approximately 10,000 taste buds with receptors for salty, sweet, bitter, sour, and umami (savory) flavors. Every time you eat food that you like, the receptors for that flavor get stimulated and send signals to your brain's pleasure centers. The receptors are active, and that's why you like eating what you like eating.

The average lifespan of a human taste bud is seven to ten days. In other words, every week or so, you will grow new cells with new receptors. If you can avoid stimulating that particular flavor with which you struggle for only one week, you will regenerate new cells with different active receptors, and as a result, you will develop new favorite flavors. That's why going cold turkey is usually the most effective approach, because once you survive the initial tough period of seven to ten days, you will thrive and lack all cravings for your previous favorite foods.

In contrast, if you transition slowly and gradually, you stimulate the taste receptors from time to time and just enough to remind the pleasure centers in your brain what you are hooked on. Then each time you refrain from your addictive food, you feel deprived and you struggle. Eating healthy whole foods is not motivating because your taste buds are not accustomed to them and thus they don't taste as good. While some people can do it gradually, if you have problems, make up your mind to go cold turkey for just two weeks. Afterwards, it will become easy and self-motivating. Or, shall we say go cold kale?

[26]

MAINTAINING AN ALKALINE BODY

WHY IT MATTERS

An athlete with an overly acidic body will recover more slowly and consequently will experience fatigue. As with any stressor, the acidity will cause the cortisol levels to rise, which will impair sleep and make the problem worse. A sleep-deprived athlete has high cortisol levels and produces lower amounts of the growth hormone, which causes a loss of muscle mass and an increase of the fat tissue.

To correct this, the frustrated athlete starts training harder, but without a proper recovery, and the vicious circle begins. Additionally, metabolic acidosis causes kidney stones and loss of bone mass. Since it affects the body at a cellular level, it increases the production of free radicals and decreases the production of cellular energy. Many viruses and bacteria thrive in an acidic body and increase the risk for various diseases. In contrast, in an alkaline body not even cancer can develop.

Unfortunately, many athletes are used to eating processed protein bars full of preservatives and other chemicals, drinking sugary sports drinks, or consuming loads of processed protein powders in a false faith of improving performance. These "sport supplements" are highly acid-forming and in that sense, almost as bad as grabbing a soda, a candy bar, or a bag of chips.

Acid-forming nutrition is detrimental to anybody's health, but especially to athletes. An overly acidic body negatively affects performance, prolongs recovery, decreases the intensity of training, and increases the risk of injury. Paying attention to the alkaline-acidic balance, (optimizing the body's performance at the cellular level by maintaining an alkaline environment) will dramatically increase athletic performance.

Your body and performance depend upon the health of your cells. You need to maintain proper pH (potential hydrogen) levels to maintain good cellular health. On the pH scale, seven is neutral, any level below is acidic, and any level above is alkaline.

Chemical processes are the most efficient at an ideal pH. The body functions the best in a slightly alkaline state. Blood has a pH of 7.4 and dipping below 7.2 pH results in death. To avoid death, your body will do whatever it takes to neutralize acidic waste and maintain homeostasis, even if it means stealing the alkaline materials (calcium, magnesium, potassium, sodium, iron) from the surrounding tissues and bones. While the body has its own smart buffering system (kidneys and lungs) to neutralize the acidic waste, sometimes it is not enough.

These buffering systems are taxed and depleted by diets overabundant in meats, dairy, processed grains, sport drinks, sodas, and other processed foods, most prescription drugs, artificial sweeteners and synthetic vitamin and mineral supplements, mental stress, performance anxiety, environmental toxins, and large amounts of acidic waste from frequent high-intensity training. When the buffer reserves are all empty, in attempt to buffer the acidic waste, the body will pull out the alkaline minerals from the bones and connective tissue, leaving them more prone to injuries such as strains, fractures, and other chronic overuse injuries.

The more energy the body spends on cleaning the acidic waste, digesting processed and overly cooked foods that lack digestive enzymes and nutrients, the less energy will be left for intense training and recovery.

The paradox of the athlete is that they eat large amounts of food and usually pay attention to their protein intake, which they believe should be high. They are used to eating commercial protein bars, powders, and shakes, which are highly acid forming, but to aid the recovery and to nourish the body, it is extremely important to consume highly alkalizing foods immediately after exercise.

The good news and solution to this paradox is that eating whole foods plants and choosing those with higher amounts of protein will deliver adequate amounts of protein, covering the athletic needs efficiently.

SPECIFIC RECOMMENDATIONS

Raw hemp protein, natural and unprocessed, contains about 50% protein (calculated per calorie, not weight) and is less acid forming than other processed proteins such as whey or soy. Hemp has high amounts of chlorophyll that is responsible for the alkaline characteristic and its green color.

Other highly alkalizing protein sources are chlorella, which contains nearly 70% protein, spirulina with over 60% protein, and green peas with about 30% of protein. A good rule for raw, whole, and unprocessed plants is that the greener they are (more chlorophyll), the more alkalizing they are. Many of the alkalizing vegetables have surprisingly high amounts of protein.

Alkalizing vegetables	Protein %
Chlorella	70%
Spirulina	60%
Hemp	50%
Spinach	49.7%
White mushrooms	31%
Green peas	28.7%
Broccoli	27.2%
Iceberg lettuce	25.7%
Green beans	21.6%
Tomato	19.6%
Celery	17.3%
Cucumber	17.3%
Corn	13.4%
Onions	12.4%
Potato	10.8%
Carrots	8.7%

Eating many green leafy vegetables will support alkalinizing of your system even during the most intense training phases. Other good sources of alkalizing protein are sprouted lentils, beans, peas, seeds, and rice. Making a smoothie with green leafy vegetables and some hemp protein after your training session will deliver optimal nutrition for a speedy recovery.

START YOUR DAY RIGHT

After a night of fasting, a good way to start your day is to build up the bodily stores of bicarbonate and alkalizing minerals. Drink a glass of water with all these items:

1. two tablespoons of apple cider vinegar or lemon juice (lemon juice and apple cider vinegar, even though they taste acidic, produce an alkalizing ash when digested)

2. a half teaspoon of baking soda (aluminum-free)

3. one tablespoon of blackstrap molasses (blackstrap molasses is the most nutritious food for high amounts of the alkalizing minerals such as iron, calcium, potassium, magnesium, and manganese, all essential for a healthy body and athletic performance)

4. optional: add a half teaspoon of sea salt (not the highly processed table salt) into your glass for even higher potency

---

Paying attention to the alkaline environment will not just improve your performance, but your health and wellbeing. Whole foods plant-based nutrition makes maintaining the alkaline-acidic balance much easier for the following reasons:

1. All of the animal products and dairy are acidic, and we don't eat them anymore.

2. Most of the processed foods are acidic, which is the reason that we don't eat them anymore.

3. All oils are acidic, but we don't eat them anymore, or only very little.

4. Most of the vegetables and fruits are alkaline, and we eat a lot of them.

It is evident that eating a whole foods plant-based diet makes life easier from many different aspects. There are several different pH balance charts available on the internet, and they all vary slightly because of the way food pH is measured. I am not going to list the complete charts because for the plant-based whole foods athlete, things are much simpler. I will only list the few acidic plants to be aware of, to make sure you are not overeating them regularly. When you do eat them, always make sure that you eat many of the alkaline plants in addition to them.

THE RIGHT BALANCE AND TREATING YOUR WATER

Most vegetables and fruits are alkaline-forming. The recommendations are to eat about 70–80% of alkaline-forming foods and 20–30% acid-forming foods. Eating whole foods plant-based nutrition matches these numbers impeccably. Drinking plain water rather than acid forming sport drinks is crucial, but unfortunately even plain water often is too acidic because it lacks the alkalizing minerals and instead contains contaminants such as fluoride and chlorine.

The recommended pH levels for water are 7.5–9.5. There are alkaline and ionized products on the market to increase hydration, but you can create your own alkaline water with much less expense by adding a plain sodium bicarbonate (baking soda). Always use aluminum-free baking soda. Depending on your water supply, you may need to use one-half to one full spoon of sodium bicarbonate per one quart of water to make it slightly alkaline. To make things more precise, buy pH sticks (online, hardware, or pool and spa stores carry them) that will measure the pH levels of your water by immersing in it, and experiment how much baking soda you need to add to make your water alkaline. Many top athletes believe that the alkaline water enhances their endurance, power, and recovery because their bodies buffer the metabolic waste with a higher efficiency, which improves the nutrient absorption and utilization.

THE BLACK SHEEP: THE ACIDIC PLANTS IN THE ALKALINE PLANT WORLD

ACID-FORMING VEGETABLES AND LEGUMES

Asparagus tips (white), beans (all dried), Brussels sprouts, garbanzo beans aka chickpeas, lentils, and rhubarb.

ACID-FORMING FRUITS

All fruits that are preserved, jellied, canned with sugar, dried with sulphur, and glazed; cranberries, green tipped bananas, olives (green or pickled), and raw fruit with sugar.

ACID-FORMING GRAINS AND CEREALS

Almost all grains, besides amaranth, millet, buckwheat, wild rice, and quinoa.

ACID-FORMING NUTS AND SEEDS

Brazil nuts, cashews, peanuts, pecans, tahini, walnuts; butters from all these nuts, more so if they are roasted.

The few alkaline-forming nuts are almonds, chestnuts, and coconut.

ACID-FORMING SWEETENERS

All chemically processed sweeteners such as Nutrasweet, Equal, Aspartame, Sweet-n-low; processed honey, molasses, white sugar, and brown sugar.

Alkaline-forming sweeteners are Stevia, rice syrup, maple syrup, raw honey, and raw sugar.

ACID-FORMING BEVERAGES

All alcoholic drinks, coffee, sodas and soft drinks, black tea, and vinegar.

Alkaline-forming beverages are herb teas, lemon water, green tea, and ginger tea.

OTHER ACID-FORMING THINGS

All drugs, aspirin, candies, cocoa and chocolate, condiments (salt, pepper, curry, spices), dressings and thick sauces, preservatives, anxiety , lack of sleep, stress, tobacco, and too much work.

It is apparent that it is much easier to maintain an alkaline environment in the body when eating a whole foods plant-based diet because nearly all vegetables and fruits are alkaline, and juices and sprouts are highly alkaline. The most alkaline-forming juices are fig juice, green juices of all green vegetables and tops, carrots, beet, celery, pineapple, and citrus juices. In addition, vegetable broth is an extremely alkalizing drink.

Paul Chek, a holistic exercise specialist, summarizes the elements of athletic performance with simple, yet remarkable words:

"The best drug for your performance is
vegetables, fruits, water, sleep,
and a reason to be alive."

SECTION 4

FOOD PREPARATION

[27]

MICROWAVE OVENS: TO USE OR NOT USE?

There are two opposite pools of opinion on the microwave oven's dangers or innocence. To this day, there are no final and clear conclusions. Until we get clear results, I believe it is better to be on the safer side. The following facts and study results will help you to make a conscious decision.

Back in 1976, the Soviet Union banned microwave ovens because they discovered that every microwave oven leaks harmful radio waves and anyone within ten feet of the microwave oven had measurable cellular damage. It is astonishing that despite these results, 90% of Americans own a microwave oven at home or work these days. Most restaurants have at least a few. While all other forms of cooking create heat from the outside in, the microwave oven is the only one that creates heat from inside out, with the friction of the pulsating radio waves.

In 1991, there was an unfortunate tragedy of death followed by a lawsuit, where Ms. Norma Levitt received a blood transfusion where the blood was heated to the body temperature level in a microwave oven. This tragic situation makes us aware that there is much more to heating and cooking with microwave oven than we may understand. Studies show that people consuming microwaved milk and vegetables had decreased hemoglobin levels and overall white blood cell levels, while the cholesterol levels increased. The greatest increase in cholesterol levels was after consuming microwaved vegetables.

Many modern families cook everything in their microwave ovens such as water, oatmeal, vegetables, meat, rice… nearly everything. Microwaves alter the nutritional profile of foods. They completely eliminate the essential food enzyme, which assist in food digestion and absorption of all the vital nutrients. Without enzymes in foods, there is no nutritional value. Eating overcooked foods without enzymes causes cell damage and has cancerous effects on the blood, more so for microwaved foods than for any other style of food preparation.

Another problem with microwaving foods is the newly formed radiolytic compounds produced by molecular decomposition from the radiation. These unusual unions don't exist in nature, and we are not sure if they are safe to eat. One study showed that microwaving vegetables destroyed up to 97% of their nutritional value. Additionally, various minerals in vegetables were altered into cancer-causing free radicals. Minerals such as calcium, magnesium, and zinc are usually not affected by microwaving, but many other necessary nutrients such as B vitamins, vitamin C, vitamin E, anthocyanins and flavonoids (powerful antioxidants), and other nutritional elements are quickly destroyed, leaving the vegetables "nutritionally dead."

For an athlete, eating nutrient-empty foods is expressed by a lack of energy, slow recovery, and a chronic inflammation that causes injuries. The combination of eating nutritionally empty foods and being exposed to various environmental stressors creates a tremendous burden on the body.

People eat too many calories because the body craves the nutrients, but the nutrient-empty foods only deliver excess calories without the healthy nutrients. These large amounts of dead food overburden the digestive system, which results in digestive problems, obesity, diabetes, heart disease, depression, liver and kidney disorders, autoimmune disorders, and many other diseases.

Both women and men who eat microwaved foods have disturbed hormone production and unstable hormonal balance. People exposed to microwave emission fields have significantly higher levels of brainwave disturbance, causing decreased concentration, memory loss, disturbed sleep, and decreased mental processing. Today's people are the sickest, and a big part of it is that they eat processed and dead foods.

I made my decision to abandon my microwave oven in early 2000s. For a couple of weeks, while I still owned it, I tried to ignore it while I was re-learning how to prepare my foods the "old fashioned" way. The presence of the microwave oven was tempting to use when I was in a hurry or just plain lazy, so I made a radical change: I donated the microwave oven to charity. No more temptations now, and I had to figure out things in a different way. The transition back to the oven and stove is simpler than you can imagine. At first, it feels like a lot of extra work because everything takes a little longer to prepare. It is mostly because you are not experienced. Every new habit takes extra effort. Once you get used to it, the actual food preparation times are very similar. The only hassle is that there is one extra pot to wash; but it is a hassle worth having in exchange for good health.

If you use a microwave oven regularly, you may be doing a disservice to yourself, especially if you have health challenges, weight issues, and performance problems. Consider giving your microwave oven away, and eating more fresh foods instead. You will have more space on your counter top, you will feel better, and your athletic performance will improve.

During your transition to the plant-based world, you will find the beauty of eating many of your foods raw. Foods that you prefer to eat warm, you can steam quickly in a pot, roast in the oven, or prepare as a quick stir-fry. It works just as great. You will soon realize that your microwave oven is an easy object to be without, if you so choose.

[28]

COOKWARE

There are many misconceptions about the best cookware. As a plant-based athlete, you don't need to worry about burning your steak or scrambled eggs anymore, but you still want to use the right cookware to preserve as many nutrients as possible.

For any cookware, always avoid cooking at higher temperatures, because the high temperatures destroy more nutrients and compromise the integrity and safety of the cookware. To preserve the most nutrients in your foods, cook them below 200 degrees.

Cookware is very important, because many conventional styles leach heavy metals that alter food enzymes and ultimately end up stored in the body. There is no completely safe cookware but some are better than others, and some are plainly toxic.

TEFLON COOKWARE

Teflon cookware is probably the supremely worst of all. The chemical PFOA that is used in manufacturing of Teflon is found in almost everybody's blood stream in the US. According to John Hopkins Medical Center, high blood levels of PFOA in humans are associated with cancer, high cholesterol levels, thyroid disease, and compromised fertility. The Teflon surface breaks down during high temperatures and ends up in your body, and the emitted fumes cause flu-like symptoms. All PFOA has to be eliminated by 2015. Get ahead of the game and throw away all of your Teflon pans now.

ALUMINUM COOKWARE

Aluminum cookware is the most common one, but it can also be very toxic because this heavy metal is absorbed into every food that you cook in it. Excess aluminum in the body has been linked to estrogen-driven cancers and Alzheimer's disease.

COPPER COOKWARE

Copper cookware is popular because it conducts heat well. It usually has nickel in the coating, and both nickel and copper are released into the food, and can be very allergenic.

CERAMIC, ENAMEL, AND GLASS COOKWARE

Ceramic, enamel, and glass cookware are manufactured with lead. The levels of lead depend on the manufacturer, and you should never cook with anything that is labeled "for decoration only."

STAINLESS STEEL COOKWARE

Stainless steel cookware is made from a metal compound, consisting of iron and chromium with different percentages of molybdenum, nickel, titanium, copper, and vanadium. Even stainless steel can leach metals into foods. Iron, chromium, and nickel have the most adverse effect on our health.

TITANIUM COOKWARE

Titanium cookware poses the least health risks because it doesn't react with foods during cooking. However, titanium cookware is highly priced, and with price tags well above $100, is not affordable for everyone. If you're thinking about long-term health, investing in titanium cookware may cost more now, but inferior cookware will cost more over time when you struggle with your health. If titanium cookware is out of your reach, cast iron will be the next good option.

CAST IRON COOKWARE

Cast iron cookware is very durable, has been used for many generations, and costs about $30. It will replace Teflon and toxic aluminum cookware with great success. It distributes the heat evenly, and when properly seasoned, it is easy to take care of. Cast iron cookware that is seasoned properly matches the qualities of non-stick cookware, and the food lifts easily from the pan after cooking. You can use cast iron on the stove and in the oven at any temperature for making bread, frittatas, and flat breads. Food cooks beautifully in a cast iron skillet, which heats evenly and creates a beautiful golden brown, crispy exterior on your foods.

Cast iron cookware is quite heavy and doesn't scratch, so you don't need to worry about using plastic or wood utensils. Just make sure that you season it well so it will continue to be non-stick and rust-free. It is very easy to clean up; soap is not needed or recommended. If the cookware is not properly seasoned, the iron can leach into the food and change its enzymes.

If the iron in the body reaches toxic levels, it can cause stress, nausea, vomiting, damaged intestinal tract lining, shock, liver failure, oxidation, and eventually more severe illness. However, in general too much iron (above 45 mg per day) is primarily caused through extra supplementation. Properly seasoned cast iron cookware doesn't leach significant amounts of iron and for the majority of the population cast iron will boost the intake of iron, which will increase energy levels and strengthen the immune system.

When eating whole foods plant-based nutrition, you will not need any additional supplements besides vitamin B12. In the modern western diet, the iron problem is opposite: 30–35% of Americans do not get enough of it. Iron deficiency, where the blood doesn't circulate oxygen efficiently, creates a feeling of tiredness, headaches, and in some extreme cases, anemia.

Athletes may be subject to low iron levels because about one milligram of iron a day is lost through perspiration. Excessive coffee and tea drinking may prevent iron absorption. However, if you are one of the few people who have high iron levels, you should avoid cast iron cookware.

[29]

JUICING

Drinking freshly squeezed juices has numerous health benefits. The short-term health benefits are increased energy levels and digestive relief. The long-term benefits are prevention of chronic illness, delayed and, in many cases, reversed aging, and improved overall wellbeing and performance.

The more imbalance and disease your body has, the more beneficial juicing is for you. If you acutely require significant amounts of nutrients, juicing is the way to go, because cooking and other food processing destroys the healthy micronutrients by altering their chemical composition and shape. You need to avoid all processed foods and eat organic vegetables and fruits as much as possible.

Medical professionals recommend eating six to eight servings of vegetables and fruits per day, but in reality, only a small percentage of people eat that amount. Many of those who do, either cook or microwave them, so they are not taking in the necessary nutrients after all. For maximum nutrient retention, the preferred way is to eat the vegetables and fruits raw. But can you imagine eating a huge plate full of raw vegetables? Unless you love to chew, it will be tough, and you probably won't stick with it for long.

While you are transitioning to a plant-based lifestyle and regaining your health, complementing your nutrition with fresh juices can be one of the best daily things you can do. When juicing your vegetables and fruits, you deliver far more health-promoting nutrients to your system than you would by eating them straight or preparing them in any other way. It would be very difficult to chew several pounds of raw carrots in a day, but when squeezed into a juice, you can deliver enormous amounts of vitamin A to improve your night vision, healthy skin, and to detoxify the liver. A clean liver efficiently processes all the chemicals we are exposed to daily. The liver is your fat-burning organ, and when the liver is clean, you will lose excess fat if you need to.

Add cabbage to your carrots when juicing. Cabbage protects your body from cancer, boosts your body's detoxification enzymes, and removes environmental estrogens, which can create a variety of hormone problems and stubborn belly fat.

Greens are an extremely important element in your plant-based diet, because they add a lot of chlorophyll, which is a powerful blood cleanser and blood builder. Chlorophyll has a similar structure to human red blood cells, and adding many raw (uncooked) greens into your diet will deliver the building materials required for the body to produce a lot of fresh blood. You will notice that your endurance and performance will increase after adding many raw greens.

Combining several different vegetables creates delicious flavors and guarantees adequate intake of many health-promoting vegetables that you would never eat otherwise, several times per day. If you add some sweet fruit to your glass, it will taste better than any soft drink. Soft drinks promote and create disease, while the delicious juices and shakes will create health, longevity, and increased performance.

REASONS TO JUICE

1. Most people have compromised digestion from all the years of subpar nutritional choices. The body is not capable of extracting and absorbing all the nutrients from the vegetables consumed as whole foods. Juicing will somewhat "pre-digest" the food, so you will absorb all the nutrients better. You may need less juicing when your health and digestion returns back to its powerful state.

2. The common recommendations are to eat at least one pound of raw vegetables per fifty pounds of body weight per day, which may feel like a heroic effort if you are not used to eating vegetables. Juicing makes the intake of several pounds of vegetables easy. As you get more accustomed to eating so many vegetables, you may juice less and chew more, because it's fun to chew after all. Enjoying your delicious meals while slowly chewing will become the highlight of your day.

3. We are all people of habit, who like eating the same foods all the time. If vegetables and fruits are already part of our lifestyle, the variety is probably somewhat limited. It is easy to add diversity to your diet through juices. You can be adventurous with vegetables, because even if your juice turns out somehow tasteless, you can always add a sweet fruit to the mixture and it will become yummy again. As you get used to the different flavors while receiving all the benefits of a variety of nutrients,

you will develop a habit of buying and eating many different vegetables and it will be easy to maintain that habit once you start preparing your meals in different ways. A new world of culinary deliciousness will open for you.

WHAT KIND OF JUICER?

What kind of juicer should you buy? If you have never juiced before, you may feel a bit uncertain as to whether you will like your new juicing lifestyle, and may not feel comfortable investing big money into a juicer. They range from $30 to $2,000. I would highly recommend skipping the cheapest centrifugal juicers, as they break easily, produce low juice quality, are very loud, and often are hard to clean. You get what you pay for, which in this case is so much hassle that will discourage you from juicing and enjoying the process. I had a cheap juicer before, but I was not motivated to use it and eventually donated it to the Salvation Army and purchased a better one that I love tremendously!

Unless you are already sure that you will be juicing daily and a lot, or if you have a medical condition for which you will have to juice a lot, the mid-range juicer will probably be a good start for you. Choose a masticating juicer with low RPMs. They are quieter, have a great juice yield, preserve many nutrients, and are super easy to clean. I own the Omega 8006, which is excellent, one of the best ones in the mid-range. Newer models are now available and also vertical versions. It is a personal choice, so you decide what you prefer. Other great brands are Green Star, Breville, Super Angel, Green Power, and Samson.

For an inexperienced health nut (maybe that's you?), juicing may seem like a difficult task. Once you try it a few times, you will be pleasantly surprised at how quick the process is. It is much easier than you thought. The cleaning is simple too, if you do it immediately after juicing. My Omega 8006 is clean in less than three minutes.

Keep in mind that vegetable juices are just an addition to your new plant-based nutrition. They are not staples of your food, rather just a pleasant and super-healthy snack. If you have a more serious health condition, you may need to juice more often, or perhaps all of your meals need to be juices. Once you recover your health, add the juices to the other meals when needed...your body will tell you.

When you start juicing, use the vegetables that you would normally enjoy eating raw or non-juiced. Since you are used to the flavor, you will most probably find your juice delicious. Then start adding some other "adventurous" vegetables to your juices, to increase your comfort level and the nutritional values. Add them slowly into the combination that you already like and get used to the new taste. After a while, add other new and different vegetables. You should feel energized after drinking the juice, not nauseous. If your stomach is making weird noises, it may be that one of your new additions doesn't agree with your stomach.

My favorite greens are spinach, celery, bok choy, kale, cucumber, and chard of all colors. If you are just starting with juicing, try two ounces of spinach, two pieces of celery, and an apple. You will be surprised at the mild and nicely sweet flavor of your juice. If you prefer a sweeter taste, add a tiny bit of Stevia or honey, and if prefer more sour, add lemon to your juicer.

Once you get used to the flavor of green juice, you can start adding stronger greens, such as kale, chard, and lettuce. Cucumber and cauliflower add mild flavor. Celery is surprisingly mild and earthy. Finally, you can add other vegetables such as carrots, beets, cabbage, broccoli, and mustard greens. Play with adding some spices: anise, ginger, turmeric root, parsley, mint, or cilantro. Only your imagination sets the limits. Well, your taste buds too, but they will get used to the new tastes quickly. Always remember that adding a sweet fruit, such as apple, apricot, nectarine, pear, pineapple, mango, and berries, makes any vegetable juice taste excellent.

After you master a perfect juicing technique, you still may find juicing somewhat time demanding. At times, when you feel rushed, you may want to juice in bulk to save yourself some work and cleaning. Just be aware that the enzymes and phytochemicals are highly sensitive to oxygenation, and their nutritional value will diminish over time. Always drink your juices as fresh as possible. If you really need to save your juice for later, you can store it up to 24 hours if you do it carefully. Store it in an airtight jar with minimum possible air left to prevent oxidizing. As long as you remove the air from the jar by vacuum sealing it, your juice will remain fresh for up to 24 hours.

A note worth mentioning: it is better to drink a slightly aged juice than no juice at all or, even worse, a sugary soda. Don't stress about the freshness if your lifestyle doesn't allow you to create freshly squeezed juice each time you need it.

Remember to clean your juicer immediately after you are done with the extraction or you will regret it multiple times later. A dried up juicer is not fun to clean. Even cleaning a freshly used cheap juicer can be a chore, but a quality juicer is clean in less than three minutes. Make sure your juicer is cleaned extremely well so mold doesn't develop and contaminate your future drinks.

CREATIVE AND HEALTHY USES OF THE JUICE PULP

The next question for the juicing beginner is what to do with all the pulp, the delicious fiber extracted from your plants. Since I always feel bad throwing away any food, I tend to be creative and do something edible and yummy with it.

1. Add spices that you like, such as pepper, oregano, cumin, marjoram, salt, and create patties from the pulp, which you can bake in the oven or prepare in the dehydrator to eat later.

2. Compost the pulp.

3. Add some pulp to your pet's bowl. They will benefit from the extra fiber as well.

4. Sprinkle it on salads; add to guacamole, stews, or soups.

5. Make a veggie broth for soups and freeze it in small servings.

6. Create vegetable crackers and bake them in the oven or dry them in the dehydrator. Similar to the veggie pulp patties, add your favorite spices and some seeds, such as sesame, chia, or flax seeds, and shape thin "patties" that will dry thoroughly and become beautifully crunchy and delicious. The pulp cracker is my favorite late night snack because it is low in calories, high in fiber, and very satisfying.

7. Add spices and make a spread for your bread or potatoes.

8. Add some of it back into your juice to make it thicker and more filling.

9. Add it to your baking, such as carrot cake, zucchini bread, or apple muffins. It will make them moist, healthy and you don't need to use any fat.

10. Make bread with added pulp for moisture and fiber.

11. Personally, I love the pulp from apples and carrots, mixed with a bit of lemon juice, honey, or Stevia, adding some water for more moisture, and topped with a few raisins and walnuts. It is the most amazing raw snack you can imagine.

TWO NEGATIVES OF JUICING

We have addressed the many benefits of juicing, but the opponents of juicing have a few valid arguments as well. The standard western diet already contains insufficient amounts of fiber, and now we are extracting the fiber from the vegetables. This is a good point, but we don't need to discard the fiber. We can use it to create other meals from it. I believe that it is so much better to consume several pounds of vegetables and fruits in the form of juice than not eating them at all. A person on a standard western diet cannot even imagine eating one third of a plate of vegetables, so how would they handle eating several pounds?

Another valid argument is ingesting too much sugar. If you make your juices mostly from fruits—and yes, they do taste delicious—then your sugar intake is most likely much higher than it should be. If you have diabetes or problems with your blood sugar, you need to be aware of this and be careful. However, this is easy to fix. Always make sure that the foundation of your juice is vegetable-based with many green leaves and only add fruits (or just one fruit) as flavor enhancers to make it fruity and sweet.

Not that bad, compared to all the positives, right?

JUICE IS THE CHERRY

Lastly, let us remember that juicing should not be the staple of your diet. Grains, legumes, vegetables, and fruits in their original chewable form are the foundation, and juices are the cherry on top.

For athletes, recovery after exercise is one of the major determining factors of athletic success. Reducing the recovery time between your workouts will make a big impact on your overall performance. Using nutrition to your advantage is something you need to think about daily. Adding more vegetables and fruits into your diet is one great step toward your athletic goal, health, and longevity.

[30]

SMOOTHIES

I love to have my vegetables and fruits blended and emulsified into a smoothie. All of the fiber remains in the smoothie, and the creation is delightfully thick and filling. I used to use the NutriBullet, a small 24-ounce monster blender, but eventually upgraded to a power blender. My new 64-ounce Vitamix makes the job much easier because it is considerably bigger and more powerful than the little NutriBullet. (Blendtec is another great high-powered blender). You throw all of your produce in, blend for 20–30 seconds and the result is a smooth texture.

Without much thinking and planning, I place into my blender whatever I find in the fridge that appeals to my eye and appetite: many green leafy vegetables, some sweet fruit, and often I add flax seeds, chia seeds, hemp seeds, nuts, or hemp protein. If the fruit is frozen, the smoothie tastes like an ice cream. During the cold weather months, I blend it a longer time to get a warmer smoothie.

My morning pre-exercise smoothie always consists of leafy vegetables and a banana for sweetness and calories. This staple makes it yummy and healthy. Then each time I use a few various additional ingredients, such as apples, pears, peaches, figs, cucumber, celery, zucchini, cauliflower, avocado, or anything that I enjoy, to give it a different flavor and nutrients. I make my smoothie about 400–500 calories and even though it doesn't seem like much, the energy that the smoothie provides is unthinkable. I can run and play tennis, or work out for a couple of hours with energy levels so high that even I am perplexed. It is not even comparable to my previous "traditional" breakfast, which was oatmeal, cereal, or a whole grain sandwich.

If it weren't for the smoothie, I would never (never ever!) eat kale, chard, or bok choy for breakfast. This was a huge revelation for me, and I love it even more each day when my physical energy is exploding. I used to wonder why this small meal delivers so much exercise vigor. All the nutrients that the body receives from the smoothie are quickly digested and go straight into the bloodstream. The digestive tract doesn't need to waste any energy on processing the food and converting it into something more energetically useful. You use all the saved energy for training instead.

During my two hours of training, I never hit the wall because of a lack of energy. I start feeling hungry when I am done. If I have to exercise longer than two hours, I make another smoothie and take it with me in a water bottle to sip during training. It works great, without any digestive or other issues. Every time I experience this "energetic indulgence" I always mutter to myself, "be blessed, my friend Kale!"

BENEFITS OF SMOOTHIES

1. A smoothie feels like a real meal. You can add any possible ingredient to make the nutritional proportions just what you want. You can even add tofu to it.

2. Thanks to the fiber content, the smoothie stabilizes your blood sugar and energy levels, because the calories are absorbed at a slow rate and the energy releases evenly, over a long time.

3. The smoothie fills you up effectively, thanks to the fiber, and you won't feel hungry for a long time.

4. They keep your digestive tract moving and thus improve regularity.

5. If you need to lose excess fat, you most probably will. The smoothie satisfies you even with a small amount of calories. You don't feel hungry, and you feel satiated without cravings. You won't be snacking, but if you need to have an extra snack, make yourself another delicious smoothie.

6. They are cost efficient. You eat everything that you blend. Compared to juicing, there is no excess pulp. Even though you can reuse the pulp from the juices, sometimes people are not able to do so at the same rate as juicing, and eventually end up throwing some of the pulp away.

7. You can get a high quality little blender (NutriBullet) for under $100. While there are other great high-powered, large blenders (Vitamix, Blendec, Ninja), the NutriBullet does an amazing job, and you will do fine with it—until it becomes too small for your needs. Oink.

8. Smoothies are quick. Your meal is ready within a few minutes.

If you can manage to both juice your plants and blend them into smoothies, go for it. That would be the ideal combination. Both have their advantages, and you can choose the right drink for the right occasion. Having more variety in your plant-based repertoire will keep you motivated and focused.

[31]

DEHYDRATING OF FOODS

When the water from the foods is removed, the taste is deliciously concentrated. Sometimes the dehydrated food tastes much better than the original, with all of the health properties retained.

You can dehydrate vegetables, fruits, and herbs. Meat-eating people make their own jerky, but plant-eating people can create delicious, healthy crackers and snacks, raw "cookies", or energy bars. It is simple, fast, and definitely much healthier and cheaper than the commercial variations.

In contrast to canning and freezing, dehydration of your foods doesn't destroy the vital nutrients such as the levels of carbohydrates, fiber, potassium, magnesium, selenium, sodium, vitamin C, vitamin A, and others. When you dehydrate your own foods at home, you can make sure that your foods are without additives and pesticides. You can control the temperature for the dehydration process and thus preserve all the nutrients.

One may consider drying the foods in the oven to achieve the same results, but unless you have a special oven with a dehydrating function, it won't work. The temperatures in the oven are usually too high for proper dehydration, and it is too humid as well. I highly recommend purchasing a dehydrator with a thermostat, which will make the dehydration process easy and efficient. The most popular brands are Excalibur and American Harvest (Nesco). There are many price ranges, and you can choose the perfect dehydrator that fits your needs. Just make sure it has a thermostat. A good quality dehydrator starts around $60 and goes way up for the professional quality levels.

You can purchase fruits and vegetables that are in season very cheaply at the local farmers' markets and whatever you don't finish eating, dehydrate and store safely for a long time. You can use canning jars for storing the dehydrated snacks, but be aware, they don't last very long. They are so good to snack on.

My favorite snack is a sweet potato, which you can dehydrate without any spices. Just slice the sweet potatoes thinly and put them in the dehydrator for 16–24 hours. Other delicious sweet vegetables or fruits are carrots, apples, pears, peaches, bananas, figs, and more. You will have a crunchy and super healthy snack at your hands when you need it.

You can also rehydrate the dehydrated vegetables, fruits, and herbs in water, broth or other liquids, and use them in regular cooking. Soak them for 30–60 minutes before use. Some very thinly cut veggies or fruits require only 15 minutes. Don't soak them longer than two hours or you will lose too much of the taste and nutrition.

I was curious to see if the dehydrator really works as it promises and if it indeed preserves the healthy nutrients in the foods. I sprouted garbanzo beans until the tail came out, then I dehydrated them, and later I rehydrated them again. Afterwards, I let them sprout again. And yes, indeed, they did sprout! It proves that all of the enzymes were preserved during dehydration.

The dehydrated foods take much less space (nearly one sixth of the original food) and so you can store them easily after buying produce in bulk. They are light and easy to bring with you when you travel, or carry them in your bag as a snack for your daily work or fitness routines.

Make your own raw breads, cookies, granola, and crackers. The dehydrator creates a great consistency in some plant-based recipes such as veggie or lentil loafs, veggie and seed crackers, or deserts such raw brownies and raw banana or carrot cakes. Now you can snack without guilt.

You can create delicious, healthy snacks instead of the commercial ones. If you enjoy crunchy snacks, create your own kale chips, flax crackers, sweet potato chips, regular potato chips, and carrots. If you have a sweet tooth, dehydrate bananas, strawberries, nectarines, mangoes, apricots, pears, and other sweet fruits. You can even try dehydrated garbanzo beans sprinkled with cinnamon and Stevia. Yum.

DEHYDRATING TEMPERATURE IS CRUCIAL

If you like eating raw plants and food, you will love the dehydrator even more. When you prepare the foods at temperatures below 118 degrees Fahrenheit (47 Celsius), which is the threshold temperature where all the nutrients and enzymes remain intact, you will enjoy all the benefits of raw vegetables and fruits. According to Dr. Edward Howell, the author of Enzyme Nutrition, temperatures above 118 degrees destroy many of the enzymes. Some enzymes are more stable at higher temperatures, but all enzymes become completely deactivated at temperatures above 140–158 degrees F (60–70 Celsius) in a moist or wet state. For denser foods, it takes longer to destroy all the enzymes.

Dehydrating at proper temperatures is crucial. If you use a temperature that is too high, you will literally overheat and cook the food, and if it is too low, your food can catch mold or bacteria. Dehydrating your food correctly involves a little science, but after some experimenting, once you know all the how's and why's, it will be an easy task.

During the dehydration process, the temperature should fluctuate slightly. The temperature needs to be low enough for the enzymes to stay alive and high enough to draw out the moisture rapidly to stop mold and bacteria from growing. When the temperature is low, it draws the moisture from the center of the food and then the moisture begins to evaporate when the temperature goes up. When all the moisture is gone, the food temperature will even out. The enzymes are destroyed only when it is hot and wet and the same time. Once the food is dry, the enzymes survive up to 150 degrees.

Inside the dehydrator, the food temperature is about 20 degrees lower than the air temperature during the evaporation process. When the dehydrator thermostat is set on 120 degrees, the food will be about 100 degrees. At one point during the dehydration process, all moisture will be gone and the food cannot develop mold or bacteria anymore. Make sure that your foods are completely dehydrated within 36 hours. If the dehydrated foods smell bad or get moldy, discard them immediately. If you have difficulty getting your foods to dry within 36 hours, either slice them into thinner pieces or lay them out in a less dense pattern for better airflow so they can dehydrate faster. Store the dehydrated foods in an airtight container in a cool place. They will remain fresh for up to one year. If you want to store your dehydrated foods longer, up to two years, vacuum-seal the canning jars or use special plastic bags.

When I started to dehydrate my foods, I was very excited and everything tasted excellent. I was crunching on sweet potatoes, dehydrated garbanzo beans, home-made crackers, and energy bars. This is not a problem because all are healthy snacks, but you need to be aware that dehydrated food doesn't have any moisture, and if you eat a lot of it, you need to drink a lot of water, so you don't get constipated. I do not have those problems as I drink 12–16 glasses of fresh water daily, but people who don't have the habit of hydrating well, should keep this in mind and drink much more fluids.

[32]

SPROUTING

Sprouts are highly concentrated natural sources of vitamins, minerals, enzymes, and amino acids (proteins). Sprouts are biogenic, meaning that the sprouting seed releases all the stored nutrients in an explosion of life and vitality so it can become a mature plant. The sprouting seed creates new life and when you eat these raw and alive foods at the peak of their nutritional value, they will provide your body with a form of "living" energy.

Sprouts have a long history, both medicinally and nutritionally. Over 5,000 years ago, ancient Chinese physicians proposed that sprouts could cure various disorders. Sprouts have always been a main staple in the diets of people of Asian descent, and continue to be to this day. You may have seen alfalfa sprouts in the stores or chia sprouts on those chia pets and chia heads that have been popular since the 1980s. Besides these well-known sprouts, you can sprout almost any seed, legume, grain, or nut.

Sprouts are inexpensive and easy to grow. They will grow in any climate, as they don't need any sunshine or soil. There is no waste in preparation of sprouts, and from only a few cents, you can grow a nutritious organic meal full of vitamins, minerals, phytochemicals, enzymes, as well as easily digestible proteins. The growing sprouts contain nucleic acid or so-called living energy. Sprouts are high in vitamins A, B-complex, C, D, E, G, K, and even U, and minerals such as calcium, magnesium, potassium, sodium, chlorine, phosphorus, and silicon. They alkalize the body and help to strengthen the immune system, fight disease, and slow down aging.

It is rather expensive to buy the full-grown sprouts, but it is extremely easy to sprout your own at home. I was resistant to try sprouting at first, but once I figured out the process, sprouting became my favorite thing in the kitchen. I bought additional sprouting kits, and now I have several different loads sprouting, so I never run out. Many websites provide the seeds, sprouting tools, and detailed information. My favorite site is SproutPeople.org but you can find sprouting tools in your local health store as well.

You can sprout almost any seed, legume, or grain. Some taste better than others and you should try them all to figure out what you like. Only buy products that have not been chemically treated or the germination rate will drop. Broken and chipped seeds also won't sprout. One ounce of dry seed equals about one cup of mature sprouts.

Sprouting is so easy that it is almost impossible to do anything wrong, unless you abuse your little green friends and don't follow the instructions. You need a wide-mouth mason jar with cheesecloth or wire mesh to cover the top. You can also buy a special sprouter, such as the Easy Sprouter, which make the sprouting process even easier. Different sprouts have slightly different processes (time to sprout) but the main procedure is the same:

1. Soak your seeds, grains, nuts, or legumes in lukewarm water for 5–12 hours until they begin awakening to life and putting out little shoots. Make sure that your seeds have enough room to expand to at least eight times their present size. Some sprouts such as alfalfa will expand a lot: three tablespoons of alfalfa will fill a quart jar. Some legumes and nuts do not expand as much.

2. Drain the sprouts and wash them 2–3 times a day. Always drain them thoroughly by shaking and spinning. It is necessary, because you don't want to get them moldy by being too wet. Between the washes, let your sprouts rest by tilting the jar upside down at a 45-degree angle so the air could circulate freely. If you use the Easy Sprouter, all this is taken care of.

3. Continue rinsing and draining for about 3–5 days until they are ready for consumption. The time for the seeds to mature will vary, depending on humidity and temperature. If you live in a hot climate, shorten the soaking times and wash your sprouts more often to keep them cool. Set the sprouts that will become green (alfalfa and other leafy sprouts) in the sun at the end of the sprouting process so they can manufacture chlorophyll. Be gentle to your sprouts, they are very tender. They refrigerate well for several days.

You can sprout almost anything. Listed are a few favorites:

→   Legumes: garbanzo, mung, black, red, or white beans, lentils, peas, soybean

→   Leafy sprouts: alfalfa, radish, broccoli, mustard, clover, fenugreek, onion, wheatgrass

→ Grains: buckwheat, bulgur, millet, quinoa, oat, barley, brown rice

→ Nuts and seeds: cashews, almonds, peanuts, flax seeds, chia seeds, sunflower, pumpkin, hemp

Nuts and seeds don't sprout like all the other sprouts, which shoot a beautiful little tail that grows more or less long. Some sprouts even get tiny leaves, but nuts show just a little bump after soaking and they are ready to eat. My favorite sprout is alfalfa. They add a lot of volume, grow fast and big, and they develop beautiful green leaves. They grow in front of your eyes and you get a lot of pleasure from watching them sprout to life… kind of like your little green kids.

You can add the sprouts to any meal, raw or cooked, sweet or spicy, add them in salads or wraps, steam them with veggies, add them raw to your meals, grind them into a paste, add them to your baking or breads, or eat them plain as a snack. They taste great in any form. Only your imagination sets your culinary limits.

The sprouting process greatly activates all the enzymes and inhibits the anti-nutrients. Enzymes make the sprouts easy to digest. In sprouts (and in other uncooked foods), all the nutrients work together in harmony for optimal use by the human body. Cooking destroys this balance and the cooked, enzyme-deprived foods create more stress on the body, which needs to provide the enzymes to properly digest the foods instead of repairing and rejuvenating the body.

Every athlete should incorporate sprouts into his or her diet to help the body conserve its vital enzymes, stimulate metabolism, support the regenerative process, and strengthen the immune system for improved performance and regeneration.

[33]

RAW FOOD

Changing to a plant-based diet is one of the best things I have done. I love how my body feels and how it performs athletically. I love the abundant energy that I have and can share with others. However, I am always searching for new ways to improve the body and mind. In my search, I came across raw food. I have tried eating raw for a few days before, and felt that there was no way I could adopt the raw food lifestyle permanently. I loved my cooked oatmeal, soups, stir-fries, and home baked treats too much. In addition, the traditional raw recipes sounded too complicated to make. I like "simple."

Then I got my hands on Ann Wigmore's books. She was a pioneer in raw food eating and using living foods to heal the body. She founded the Hippocrates Health Institute, which to this day helps people restore their health. Ann Wigmore's recipes were really simple and much easier even than cooking.

I read everything possible on raw foods and was so impressed that I decided to try another little experiment: "eating raw for one month." The results were astonishing, and now I have adopted the raw lifestyle forever. For this reason, I feel the urge to include information on raw foods in this book, as I believe that many people may go through a similar transition to mine.

While the human genome has been developing over millions of years, and the anatomically modern human over 200,000 years, they have only been cooking food for a few thousand years. Human biological and physiological requirements were set long before we started to cook food. The human species is the only one on Earth that cooks its food and feeds cooked food to its animals. They also experience disease more than any other species.

Cooking and heat changes the molecular structure of food. Proteins are denatured and cannot perform their enzymatic activities. Fats are oxidized, producing dangerous substances such as free radicals and trans-fatty acids. Starches convert to sucrose, causing excessive sugar metabolism reactions, such as high blood sugar followed by a crash and cravings. Heat destroys enzymes and vitamins, and some minerals may become unusable by the body as cooking converts them into their inorganic state. After eating a cooked meal, the body's white blood cell count increases 3–4 times in order to neutralize and expel the offending compounds. This response is similar to taking a toxic substance.

Cooked food is less digestible than raw food with two exceptions: beta-carotene in carrots and sweet potatoes, and lycopene in tomatoes (when you puree the carrots after cooking, you release even more powerful, cancer-fighting compounds). Anything that the body doesn't digest or store properly must be eliminated. Eating cooked foods produces a lot of waste and so puts a lot of stress on the elimination organs, which cannot keep up, and waste accumulates. This leads to a toxemia that can cause inflammation, decreased energy and performance, and eventually, disease.

Obviously, cooked food is not a poison that will kill you immediately after eating. But over time, little by little, it imposes a great strain on the various organs and bodily processes with an excessive waste build-up. Years and years of eating cooked food brings the tissues in constant contact with toxins and waste, causing tissue irritation, inflammation, and degeneration. The cells die at a faster rate and the organs lose their proper function. People in their 40's and 50's start developing chronic illness. Athletes in their 30's and 40's begin to lose their athletic skills, flexibility, strength, endurance, and the ability to recover. They are more prone to injuries and the vicious cycle of constant injuries begins.

The human body has an amazing capacity to tolerate years of poor eating habits with cooked and processed foods. However, it also demonstrates how much healthier we can be if we stop this abuse. Raw foods are easy to digest, provide all the nutrients that the body needs, and are almost entirely usable by the body. The body can use the saved energy for healing, recovery, and thriving.

Knowing that we have so much control over the quality of our health and performance should motivate people to consider eating more raw foods. Some people may want to eat raw foods exclusively for the maximum health and performance benefits, but if this lifestyle seems too extreme for you, adding as many raw foods to your diet as possible will make a tremendous difference. And after some time, when you feel absolutely great, you might reconsider this raw proposal.

BECOMING RAW

People don't often realize the mental, emotional, and lifestyle changes required when switching to a 100% raw food diet. Changing old unhealthy habits and replacing them with new healthy ones takes a lot of conscious effort. You have so much to learn and you have to be prepared to search for new information about your new lifestyle. You also have to unlearn many of your eating habits that you have developed since early childhood. You need to be ready for well-meaning criticism from your friends and family members who will condemn your new lifestyle because of indoctrination or a lack of knowledge.

Just as in switching from animal foods to plant-based foods, we all have our own ways of approaching change. Some people research the information ahead and transition step-by-step, and others jump in head first and learn as they go. You know your style best, but if you've had difficulties changing your eating habits in the past, you may reconsider your style now. It could be that you are not doing the best way for your eating type.

According to Victoria Boutenko, an expert in raw food nutrition, there are two main kinds of eaters—normal eaters who eat when they are hungry and stop when full, and compulsive eaters who eat more than they need or want, not because they are hungry, but for other reasons. In her book *12 Steps to Raw Foods* Victoria states:

> "I believe that only "normal eaters" can manage to stay on a raw diet combined with small portions of cooked foods without sliding into a predominantly cooked-food diet. I would like to clarify that I don't recommend that; I only share my observation that "normal eaters" would get minimal harm from eating some cooked food because they are capable of controlling their food intake. For compulsive eaters I strongly recommend a 100% raw-food diet simply because it would be considerably easier for them to maintain."

Even if you don't plan to become a raw food athlete, Victoria's idea can be a helpful solution for your transition to the plant-based diet. Don't give yourself any room for temptations. Using our will, we can often accomplish a lot, but then there are times when we feel stressed, tired, angry, lonely, depressed, or hungry and we may succumb to the temptations. If there is no room for temptation, then the transition is much easier.

If you are convinced that transitioning to a raw food diet is for you, you should begin making changes right away. The sooner you start, the sooner you can begin enjoying the benefits. Some of the reported benefits are:

→ almost limitless energy

→ reaching your optimal, lean body weight

→ clear thinking

→ deep sleep

→ healthy, disease-free body

→ no fear of disease

→ increased self-confidence

→ balanced emotions

→ a firm body

→ smooth skin

→ improved sexual function

→ clear eyesight

→ looking and feeling younger

→ thickening of hair

→ increased self-awareness

→ enhanced focus

→ improved athletic recovery

→ increased endurance

→ lack of chronic aches and injuries

WHAT TO EAT?

You can eat vegetables, fruits, seeds, nuts, grains, and legumes. The fruits and vegetables can be eaten just as they are: take a bite and enjoy. Grains and legumes need to be sprouted to activate the enzymes and deactivate the anti-nutrients, thus making them easier to digest. Nuts and seeds, while they can be eaten raw, are easier to digest when sprouted.

→ Eat your raw foods in their natural state

→ Cut them into salads

→ Grind them and make patties and loaves in the dehydrator

→ Blend them into soups or smoothies

→ Juice them into juices

There are many amazing options for delicious raw meals. The process is slightly different from what you are used to, but when you get used to it, you will find eating raw extremely simple: no complicated meals with long preparations. It will be simple, fresh, and fast.

Raw food is the best fast food.

COOKING TIPS

Make healthy raw snacks from your favorite vegetables that you can dip in hummus, guacamole, or other delicious, healthy dips. To begin with, choose vegetables that you already like, and ultimately explore some other kinds after you acquire a liking for the raw taste and consistency. Make snacks from carrot bites, string beans, cauliflower and broccoli florets, celery, zucchini, bell peppers, radishes, cucumbers, sugar snap peas, or even slices of sweet potato.

When you make a salad, expand your horizons. A salad doesn't need to mean shredded lettuce. Add dark leaves cut into small pieces into your salad, such as kale, spinach, chard, collard, mustard greens, arugula, radicchio, bok choy (Chinese cabbage), beet greens, or dandelion leaves. Enhance the flavor of your salad with thinly sliced beets, bell peppers, cauliflower, cucumbers, tomatoes, red onions, celery, radishes, sprouts, and virtually any possible vegetable you can find.

For more filling salads, add prepared (cooked or sprouted) grains and legumes such as quinoa, brown rice, millet, barley, garbanzo beans, lentils, peas, or beans of any kind. Your imagination is the limit. The possibilities of flavors of your salads are essentially infinite.

Use shredded cabbage, bean sprouts, or grated zucchini as a raw version of rice or noodles for Asian style meals.

SECTION 5

IMPORTANT NON-FOOD TOPICS

[34]

HYDRATION

Proper hydration of your body is more important than you can believe, not just for the optimal performance but also for the necessary recovery and regeneration. When the body is well hydrated, the blood is less thick and flows better, and therefore delivers all the nutrients and hormones more efficiently. The red blood cells deliver oxygen to the muscles, while the waste products such as carbon dioxide are cleaned out. Well-hydrated cells swell slightly and create an anabolic environment for the muscle tissue to repair and grow. In contrast, a dehydrated body is in a catabolic state, breaking down muscle tissue and you don't recover properly. Your performance suffers. Dehydrated cells are more acidic and prone to disease.

CHOOSE WATER TO HYDRATE

Skip all the sodas. Even the diet sodas are harmful. Many athletes think that Gatorade-like drinks are great for hydration during athletic performance, but if you examine the label carefully, you realize that they are full of sugar, additives, and even toxic chemicals. Skip these "performance" drinks. Plain water is your best option.

If you want to have some flavor in your water, add a little bit of lemon juice, cucumber, or a piece of orange. If you prefer slightly sweeter drink, add honey, blackstrap molasses, or maple syrup. For a calorie-free drink, sweeten your water with Stevia. Never ever drink commercially made drinks and juices, which are full of empty calories and nutritionally very empty. Coffee, tea, and alcohol are diuretic and dehydrate your body. If you drink these drinks occasionally, you need to increase your water intake. Don't drink them instead of water and limit them to just occasional use.

Time your water intake correctly. It's best to drink a full glass or two of water first thing in the morning, possibly with lemon juice and a tiny bit of blackstrap molasses or maple syrup. This will hydrate your system for proper functioning after the long night as the body repairs and rejuvenates itself. Don't drink large amounts of water immediately before and after a meal, because it dilutes the digestive juices. This decreased digestive power makes your digestive system work harder and less efficiently.

Eating plant-based nutrition without processed foods will add a lot of water into your body and you will feel well hydrated through the day. Every time you drink your smoothie, you are delivering needed fluids. Smoothies are great to sip on in the morning or afternoon, supplying you with instant energy, thanks to the easily digestible nutrients and liquids.

When you eat a lot of raw fresh fruits and raw vegetables, you may never feel thirsty because the raw foods are predominantly water and you get huge amounts of liquids from them. People who prefer to eat predominantly raw foods get so much water through their food that they don't need to drink any extra liquids.

When you eat cooked foods, or even worse, processed foods, the demand for water increases immediately. Processing foods, usually at high temperatures, draws the moisture out of them, while additives like sodium and other chemicals, such as MSG are added to enhance the flavor which was lost when the processing removed all the flavorful nutrients. Eating processed foods will make you thirsty and you need to drink greater amounts of water.

Unfortunately, people who eat processed foods also drink processed drinks to satisfy their thirst. These sugary soft drinks and processed juices add excessive amounts of sugar and additional chemicals to the already too-processed meal. The body's digestive system becomes overloaded and eventually compromised. Eating plant-based foods is a much better option, especially if you also make sure to add some raw meals to your eating plan.

FLUID REQUIREMENTS

At any level of fitness, dehydration leads to decreased performance. The fluid requirements depend on the training intensity, duration, and the environment temperature during the exercise. An athlete can lose two to four quarts (liters) of fluid in one hour of intense exercise in a hot climate. In comparison, a sedentary person in a cold climate loses about 1.5 quarts (liters) for the entire day. Your physical performance is compromised by as little as one percent of body weight of lost fluids. A four to five percent loss of body weight decreases the performance by twenty to thirty percent, and an eight percent loss causes mental confusion, dizziness, and heatstroke. It is crucial to be properly hydrated before the sporting activity:

1. Drink a lot of fluids in the 24 hours before training

2. Two hours before exercising drink 2 cups (480 ml) of fluids

3. Then every 15 minutes drink 2–4 oz (60–120 ml)

4. Continue hydrating during the exercise with 4-8 oz (120–240 ml) every 10-15 minutes

5. Rehydrate optimally after the activity with 2 cups (480 ml) for each pound of bodyweight lost through sweating

(Note: these numbers are suggested by the rules for optimal hydration from the Position of The American College of Sports Medicine. Always pay attention to your body and adjust the numbers to your personal needs.)

If you experience excessive urination, it may be caused by water that lacks minerals or by mineral imbalances or deficiencies in the body. Experiment by adding a tiny amount of salt to your water (it should taste better, but not too salty) and see if you urinate less. If not, add more salt until you find the optimal amount. Once you find the correct amount, you will notice that your body will feel better and you will urinate less while drinking the same amounts of water.

As mentioned in the chapter on maintaining alkalinity, plain water may be too acidic because of mineral imbalances and lack of alkalizing minerals. To alkalinize your water, add one-half to one whole teaspoon of baking soda (aluminum-free sodium bicarbonate) into one quart of water. The amounts depend on the quality of your water supply. The final pH should be 7.5–9.5.

Eating whole foods plant-based nutrition with a lot of fruits and vegetables will make it much easier to stay hydrated, because many fruits and vegetables consist of large amounts of water. Your hydration levels will stay consistent during the day even when not training.

[35]

SLEEP

Sleeping is nothing special for a plant-based athlete. Sleep is important for everybody. However, after switching to plant-based nutrition you may notice that you have tremendous amounts of energy. Most likely you will be more active and more intense in your training. You will be capable of doing many different things and feeling great at the same time. Because you will use your body more intensely, you do need to think about regeneration and rejuvenation. When you are not active, sleep time is an important period for your body to repair.

Insufficient sleep is the primary cause of decreased performance, degenerative diseases, higher stress levels, and accelerated premature aging. If you want to achieve optimal longevity and performance, you need to pay attention to your sleep. Sleep deprivation is dangerous. It has detrimental effects on the immune system, and it makes us sick in the long term.

Most people need seven to nine hours of sleep. Listen to your body and get enough sleep to promote a full recovery from your athletic endeavors. If you follow the light-dark cycles of nature, you will notice an enormous improvement in your quality of sleep and you will feel fully rejuvenated and rested, even when sleeping fewer hours.

MELATONIN—YOUR FRIEND

While vitamin D is the daylight hormone, melatonin is the nighttime hormone, with the peak production around 2 a.m. There are many benefits of melatonin. It increases levels of the growth hormone and magnifies the results of resistance training by promoting muscle growth. Melatonin kills cancer tumor cells, prevents tumor growth, and extends survival of cancer patients. (Note: people who work at night have higher than average cancer rates, and blind people have lower than average cancer rates.) Melatonin is also effective against many chronic diseases, such as high blood pressure, diabetes, irritable bowel syndrome, glaucoma, macular degeneration, and more.

Even tiny amounts of light disturb melatonin production. You should sleep in total darkness, without any safety night-lights or LCD alarm clocks. If you need to go to the bathroom, try to do it in total darkness—it can be entertaining to see in the morning what you have done. If you wake up a lot during the night or very early in the morning, your melatonin levels may be low. If you have deficiencies in melatonin, you should supplement with time-released tablets, which can maintain sufficient levels of melatonin through the night. Melatonin is not toxic.

TIPS FOR BETTER SLEEP

→ Your bedroom should be only for sleeping (and lovemaking).

→ No electronics, TVs, computers, and tablets should be in the bedroom, because excessive electromagnetic fields disrupt deep sleep.

→ Use a comfortable bed and avoid metal coil mattresses as they emit positive ions. (Note: positive ions are bad, negative ions are excellent for us. Oceans, rivers, waterfalls, and other running waters are examples of outstanding sources of negative ions). Memory foam mattress, buckwheat pillows, and cotton or silk sheets are great.

→ Keep the temperature cool and the air fresh, letting it in from outside, using plants, quality filters, and essential oils.

→ Use fans rather than air conditioners.

→ Keep your environment quiet and dark.

→ Use ear plugs if you cannot make your environment quiet any other way.

→ If there is too much light in the bedroom, the sleep hormone melatonin may not release all of its regenerative power.

→ Reading and meditating before sleep calms your mind and stimulates your brain in a positive way.

→ If you have a partner, connect with each other in a relaxing and loving way before falling asleep. Avoid discussing any sensitive issues or subjects of disagreement.

➜ Follow the cycles of nature. Serotonin levels rise when the sun is bright and decrease when it gets dark. Light stimulates activity in the body and darkness calms the body into the mode of regeneration.

➜ Eat your larger meals earlier in the day when the sun is still up and bright. Overeating with large meals three to four hours before bedtime prevents optimal release of the regenerative hormones, because your liver and pancreas are still working on digesting the large meal. If you are still hungry before sleep, eat a light snack that is easy to digest such as fresh fruit, vegetables, light soup, herbal tea, or nut milk. Pay attention to how you feel and look in the morning after a late and heavy meal compared to a light meal: tired and puffy compared to youthful and rejuvenated.

➜ Definitely avoid caffeine, alcohol, nicotine, chemicals, and preservatives before bedtime. If you can, maybe with the exception of limited caffeine, avoid them in your general diet and in life.

➜ Sometimes, dehydration fires false alarms of hunger. Drink first and then see if you are still hungry. The bodily liquids transport the nutrients into the cells and the waste out of the cells. When you are dehydrated, the adrenal glands work harder as they assist in flushing the waste products from the cells and the toxins out of the body.

➜ Wake up, eat, exercise, and go to sleep at regular times each day, if possible. Your body likes the natural rhythms and regularity.

➜ Try to relax before sleep with calming music, sauna, hot tub, massage, meditation, or journaling.

➜ Clearing your thoughts before bedtime will make a tremendous difference in the quality of your sleep.

➜ You can use calming herbs: valerian, anise, hops, chamomile, or lavender, or essential oils such as jasmine, lavender, neroli, chamomile, geranium rose, and marjoram.

➜ Light stretching or gentle yoga can be relaxing before sleep, but any strenuous exercise should be done earlier in the day, no later than four hours before bed.

SLEEP AND STRESS

The stress hormone adrenalin, also called natural speed, will highly interfere with your sleep. The stress hormone cortisol is positively affected by sleep. It follows the circadian rhythm: cortisol levels are high during the day and low while you sleep. If you have problems with your sleep, your cortisol levels rise.

Stress is a culprit in almost every health problem. Chronically heightened stress hormone levels are the number one cause of chronic disease and will accelerate premature aging. Over time, it will harm your athletic performance due to inadequate recovery and tissue regeneration.

Each time we experience stress, adrenals are stimulated, cortisol levels are heightened and we feel a short-term burst of energy, which is followed by fatigue. Often we try to stimulate the adrenals with a cup of coffee or refined sugar. We get another burst of energy, yet again followed by even deeper fatigue. The vicious cycle repeats and the signs of adrenal exhaustion show stronger. It begins with increased appetite, which turns into cravings later. You experience difficulty sleeping, followed by irritability, mental fog, and eventual lack of motivation. You gain fat, lose muscle, and start showing signs of premature aging followed by the first signs of disease.

You can stop this vicious cycle by releasing your stress regularly with deep breathing, meditation, yoga, or other pleasant ways versus self-stimulating your adrenals with coffee, energy drinks, or drugs to increase your energy to handle stress. Your body will always adapt to the stimulants and you will need to increase the doses to get the same effect. Who knows how this could finish? One of the better outcomes is the chronically exhausted adrenals and disease, but it can get much worse. Don't take the chance.

Active stress reduction and decreasing cortisol levels should be one of the main goals in your life. When you are able to maintain low stress levels, you won't need the adrenal stimulation and you will avoid the perpetual rollercoaster of highs and lows, energy and fatigue. On the contrary, you will have endless abundant energy. Two simple ways to reduce your stress levels are sleep and exercise.

If you still feel like your stress levels are high, start practicing deep breathing, similar to one that is performed in yoga: deep, slow, diaphragmatic, or learn to practice meditation. You can practice deep breathing anytime and anywhere during the day. Even a few minutes of deep relaxed breathing will have great effects on your stress levels. Control your stress, enjoy your sleep, and your athletic prowess will skyrocket.

[36]

MEDITATION

Meditation is something that everybody should master. Many people feel like they don't have time to meditate, but these are the people who need it the most. A few minutes a day is a good start. Don't feel pressured that you have to do twenty minutes or more. Maybe you will one day, but for now, every minute counts. Do not hesitate to meditate just because you don't know how and think it has to be something fancy. Meditation is one of the most powerful things you can do. It also is one of the simplest things, because you can do it anytime and anywhere. Paradoxically, it also is one of the hardest things to do, because until you learn how to do it, you will feel discomfort with your own thoughts and you will want to quit.

You will feel benefits of meditation immediately. The instant results show as relieved stress and feeling relaxed; the long-term benefits are improved focus, improved patience, stronger willpower, lowered stress levels, feeling more present and aware in your daily activities, more focused or in the zone during your sport training, improved happiness and self-control, improved memory and academic achievement. Research suggests that improved metabolism, heart rate, respiration, and blood pressure are among the many benefits of meditation.

There are many different ways to meditate, but the simplest one is to pay attention to your breath. You can do it while in your car, waiting for a bus, sitting in a restaurant, in your office, while walking or running, or at home in the shower. You can even do it for only a couple of minutes if you think you don't have time, but there is no excuse for not doing it, because everybody can find two free minutes. It is simple and quick, yet unimaginably powerful.

If you are new to meditation, the goal is to create this new habit and meditate daily, even if just for two minutes. Don't worry what kind of meditation. Don't worry about finding the perfect place or the perfect time. Make it simple. Commit to two minutes a day. If you feel great, feel free to do more, but mainly commit to two minutes. You know that you can find two minutes anytime. The hardest thing about creating new habits is sticking to them every day. To make it easier, pick a good time and a trigger. A trigger is something that you already do regularly, and you just link your new habit to it. For example, meditate after your drink your coffee, brush your teeth, walk your dog, eat lunch, stretch after your sport activity, or when you come home from work or school. The time doesn't need to be exact, just link the meditation to the trigger event.

Find a quiet area, maybe in the early morning when nature is waking up and before everybody in the house gets up, or in the peaceful park during your lunch break. Find a place that you like and where you won't be bothered for a few minutes. If it happens that you get disturbed, don't worry, it will just strengthen your meditation.

HOW TO MEDITATE

→ Make yourself comfortable. Sit in a chair, on a bench, on the floor, or you can even lie down if you cannot sit comfortably. Lean toward a wall or tree if you have flexibility problems and cannot sit comfortably on your own. Keep your legs straight or crossed, or sit on a pillow. There are no rules.

→ Keep your eyes closed or opened.

→ Focus on your breath. When you breathe in, feel your breath through your nose, moving into your throat, then to your lungs and abdomen. When you breathe out, feel your breath leaving the body the same way. You can also visualize that you are breathing in joy and breathing out anxiety. Breathe in health and breathe out disease. Breathe in faith and breathe out worry. If your mind starts wandering, just pay attention to it and return to your breath.

Start with only two minutes. You are trying to develop a new, pleasant habit. If you jump into a 20-minute meditation that makes you uncomfortable, you will definitely not continue and maintain your habit. If you meditate for a week without skipping, try to prolong your meditation to five to seven minutes. After two weeks of uninterrupted daily meditating, increase to ten minutes. After three weeks, increase to fifteen minutes and if you were able to stick to it for the entire month, try twenty minutes. At this point, your new habit is probably established, and since you feel the great benefits of meditation by now, it will be easier to continue.

You may find the first attempts to meditate very difficult. It is hard to focus, your thoughts are racing, and you may feel uncomfortable. Don't worry. Just return to your breath. Let the thoughts race. With time, you will become better at letting them pass like a white fluffy cloud in the sky on a sunny day.

Being able to sit and pay attention to your breath is a great practice of mindfulness. You teach yourself to focus your attention, which will be extremely helpful in life and the sporting field. When you have been practicing meditation for a while, you can expand your practice to some other areas of your life:

➔ When you drive and feel the stress of the traffic, go back to your breath and pay attention to how your body feels and to the surroundings, and you will feel instantly calmer.

➔ When you eat, focus on your food, how it feels to eat, how it tastes, focus on the sensations in your mouth and your body. Feel how the food energizes you.

➔ When you feel stressed out or overwhelmed, begin to pay attention to your breath and bring your mind to the present moment.

➔ When you cook or clean, try to make every movement mindfully. Pay attention to your breath and to how your body feels in motion.

During your athletic performance, during the intense or stressful moments, always go back to your breath and you will notice soon that you will be able to enter the zone—the moments of relaxed, non-thinking, excellent performance—more frequently and almost on demand.

There are many different kinds of meditation and you can try each of them and find which one you like the best. You can combine them and use them all.

➔ Transcendental meditation focuses on a mantra—a word, sound, or phrase—that you repeat during or between every breath.

➔ Mindfulness meditation focuses on your breath and your experience during the meditation, observing your thoughts and sensation without judgment. Use this meditation when you don't need to focus, for example swimming and listening to the sound of the bubbles, walking in the park and feeling the ground under your feet, listening to the birds or wind.

➔ Sensory meditation focuses on forming mental images of things, places, or situations that you find relaxing.

➜ Personal meditation focuses on your breath while playing relaxing music, lighting a candle, playing nature sounds of rain, waves, thunder, birds, and similar. You can find many smart phone apps for meditation or guided imagery.

There are too many positive benefits of meditation to ignore it. If you feel skeptical, the only way to know is to try it. Give it one month of mindful practice and see for yourself. I am confident that you won't be disappointed.

[37]

BE GRACEFUL WITH OTHERS

Living a plant-based lifestyle can present challenges at times. Finding good plant-based food when you travel is a minor problem compared to certain social situations where you will be confronted in your interactions with meat-eaters. While some people will be curious about your lifestyle, asking many questions and becoming genuinely excited and motivated, you will find also many negative, defensive, or even very aggressive people.

Since eating whole foods plant-based diet has such a positive impact on your health and sport performance, you will feel very excited. The side effects of your new lifestyle, mainly the improved environment and wellbeing of animals, will make you feel empowered, and you will want to share your experience eagerly with everyone around you. You have to remember that when you talk about your journey, you will directly or indirectly challenge many people's lifelong beliefs and this can make them uncomfortable and sometimes even angry. Your behavior in these situations will either ruin your efforts to educate people or create marvelous success. Always honor your nutritional (and ethical) principles but do not judge, criticize, or even insult other people's values, regardless of how much you disagree with them. And that is not always easy!

Some people will respect or even admire your decision and become curious about your lifestyle, while others will feel threatened no matter what you say and how nice and polite you are. During these negative confrontations with other people, keep your mind open and try to understand why this person is reacting so strongly toward you. Never take the attacks personally, because most of the time it is about the person's insecurities and not about you. When he hears your words, he may compare himself to you and feel forced to examine his choices, which can feel very uncomfortable. In this case, it is much easier to be aggressive rather than deal with his own issues. If you handle situations like this with politeness and tact, you will keep your self-respect and peace of mind. As with any other skill in life, arts, sports, or human behavior, you need to practice it regularly until it becomes automatic.

When you talk about your plant-based lifestyle with other people, present your personal commitment to health and lifestyle confidently, but do not make other people feel bad just because they eat differently. Don't make it sound like "I am good, and you are bad." Deep inside, many people want to do the right things, but they may not have the knowledge to do so, or their living situation doesn't allow for it at the present moment. Rather than judging them, which makes them resentful and defensive, patiently talk about your views and reasons and you may be able to plant a seed in their mind. Put yourself in their situation and feel how the words you speak would affect them.

Patience and empathy go much further than pushiness and judgment. When people feel understood, they are more open to new ideas and change. We all have different journeys in this life. People are at various stages of their journeys and even a small change will be a positive change in the right direction. For example, instead of judging a person for eating a fatty hamburger, praise them for adding more vegetables to their diet. Praise them for replacing dairy with nut milks. Inspire them to make more positive changes. If you want people to cross over to your side of the plant-based river, build the bridge with kindness rather than burning it with judgments.

The best tool for persuasion is to be an example. Become a walking billboard for health and radiance, with no signs of common health problems such as high blood pressure, diabetes, or high cholesterol. Share your experience on how the plants help you to recover quickly, and how it improves your performance, without any chronic pain and injuries. Rather than convincing people how great the plant meals taste, cook a nice meal for them and let them taste for themselves. When you are walking proof of radiant health, you will remove all doubts about the benefits of a plant-based diet. Radiate the best of you in everything you do. Keep spreading the knowledge and reverence for life.

APPENDIX

NON-RECIPES

aka

RECIPE BLUEPRINTS

The premise of this book was "simple." This simple guide should help you transition with ease into the plant-based world to achieve health and maximum performance. Even though I don't follow recipes—I prefer to create my own culinary plant-based art—I often search online for recipes to get ideas for creating easy, quick, delicious, and nutritious plant-based meals.

This guide is not meant to be a cookbook. There are many great cookbooks on plant-based nutrition out there: cooked, raw, low fat, or gluten-free, and a few of my favorites are listed in the bibliography section. If you enjoy cooking and preparing elaborate meals, please, refer to the "real" cookbooks.

The following food preparation approaches are for people who want to eat nutritious foods that require little time to make. They are very simple. I call them "non-recipes" or blueprints, as you can customize them to your taste. They all take less than 15 minutes to prepare. You would spend much more time ordering a meal from a local restaurant.

Since a plant's taste varies, depending on the location and season of the year, a meal made from the same ingredients can have a different taste. Therefore, I encourage you to experiment with the final product and fine-tune the taste with spices to satisfy your taste buds. Be adventurous. Play with your foods— something that your parents maybe stopped you from doing when you were little. As you become more experienced, you will become a great, intuitive cook, creating your own delicious meals without any need for recipes.

You can also make substitutions in your meals, such as creating a soup from a salad recipe by blending it in a high-powered blender. Smoothie recipes can be left unblended and enjoyed as salads. You can thicken a soup with grains and create patties or loaves. Let your taste buds and your supply of ingredients guide your culinary adventures. The measurements of ingredients are guidelines only and you don't need to follow any recipe exactly. The lists of fruits and vegetables are far from complete.

SMOOTHIE BLUEPRINT

For the smoothest smoothie, I recommend a high-powered blender, which will thoroughly emulsify all the items, including the fruit seeds. A regular blender will work too, but the consistency may not be as perfect. Add one or two items from each group in 2 cups of liquid.

INGREDIENTS

Liquid: 2 cups
Water, tea, or nut milk

Soft fruit
Banana or ½ avocado

Fresh or frozen sweet fruit: 1 cup or 1 fruit
Berries, peaches, mango, nectarine, pineapple, pear, orange, grapefruit, or apple

Leafy vegetables: 1 cup
Spinach, chard, kale, arugula, bok choy, or lettuce

Other vegetables: 1 cup
Celery, cauliflower, cucumber, zucchini, red beet, carrot, or sweet potato

Fats: 1 oz (optional)
Any nut or nut butter, flax seeds, chia seeds, coconut oil, flax seed oil, or hemp seeds

Protein powder: 1 oz (optional):
Hemp, sunflower, pumpkin, pea, brown rice, or soy

Sweetener (optional): to taste
Stevia, honey, maple or agave syrup, dates, or raisins

Thickener (optional):
Chia seeds, flax seeds, avocado, oats, almond flour, or ice

Spices and herbs (optional):
Cinnamon, cayenne pepper, parsley, mint, basil, ginger, turmeric root, or lemon juice

Superfoods (optional):

Chlorella, spirulina, maca powder, super greens, cacao nibs, carob chips, lucuma, probiotics, blue-green algae, or Aloe Vera

DIRECTIONS

1. Put all ingredients in a high-powered blender, with the liquid first, then from the hardest to the softest item.

2. Start on the lowest speed and increase slowly to the maximum speed. Blend for another 15–30 seconds or until your smoothie looks emulsified.

3. If you enjoy the texture of wet, gooey chia seeds, add one tablespoon of chia seeds at the end when your smoothie is fully blended. Mix them in and let them swell for 5–10 minutes. They will make your smoothie thicker and chewier.

STIR-FRY, STEW, OR SOUP BLUEPRINT

The basic blueprint is the same for a stir-fry, stew, and soup. The only difference is the amount of liquids. The stir-fry has none, while the soup has the most. Preferably, cook the meal as little as possible to preserve many of the beneficial nutrients.

Make sure that you have all five flavors included in your meal: sweet, salty, sour, bitter, and spicy. Only then will the meal be satisfying and feel complete. Tweak the final concoctions with spices and flavorings to get the taste just right. With a little practice, you will learn how to balance the flavors just perfectly.

Vegetables should be the foundation of your meal, so use at least 2 cups per person. I personally prepare several pounds for myself. When you get used to the delicious flavors of the plants, you will probably eat large amounts as well, and with gusto. The combinations and options are unlimited. Add one or more items from each group.

INGREDIENTS

Vegetables:
Carrots, spinach, kale, broccoli, cauliflower, zucchini, onions, bok choy, peas, turnip, collard greens, green beans, celery, mushrooms, mustard greens, asparagus, eggplant, water chestnuts, radishes, cabbage, potatoes, sweet potatoes, tomatoes

Protein:
Beans and lentils of all types and colors (cooked or sprouted), tofu, tempeh, nuts, seeds, and vegan "meat" products

Spices:
Salt, pepper, garlic, curry, garam masala, parsley, cilantro, mint, scallions, soy sauce, vinegar, limejuice, sweet and sour sauce, Tabasco sauce, oregano, marjoram, turmeric

Flavorings:
Raisins, dried mulberries, goji berries, shredded coconut, tiny amounts of your favorite fresh or dried fruit

DIRECTIONS

1. Heat a cast iron pan or pot for the soup, while you are cutting all the vegetables into small pieces.

2. Sauté onion and garlic together with salt and pepper. Either use a tiny amount of coconut oil, or do the oil-free method (use one-half to one cup of water and cook on medium heat, stirring occasionally until the water evaporates. If the food is still not done, add some more water and keep going). Sauté and stir for a few minutes.

3. Keep cutting your vegetables, starting from the hardest ones to the softest ones.

4. Add the vegetables into the pan as you cut them.

5. Save the green leafy veggies and the crunchy ones until the end.

6. Finally, add all the spices and protein items, and sauté for another minute or two.

You get an amazing harmony of colors and flavors that will tease your taste buds a different way each time you create a new stir-fry. For a stew, add desired amount of water after sautéing the onions and garlic. The amount of water will depend on the vegetables you use—some will release more liquid, some less. Adjust the thickness as you progress in your meal preparation. For a soup, use even more water, depending on how thick you like your soup. The remaining process is the same.

RAW CHOWDER BLUEPRINT

This soup is raw, but you can make it warm as well.

INGREDIENTS

Base:
1 cup cashews, macadamias, or walnuts
2 cups water
2 tbsp olive oil (optional)
2–3 pitted dates
1 cup celery
1–2 cloves garlic
Sea salt, pepper, hot peppers (optional) to taste

Flavorings:
Dulse flakes (will taste like clam chowder), broccoli, mushrooms, tomato, carrots, corn, or peas

DIRECTIONS

1. Blend 1 cup of nuts with 1 cup of water in the power-blender until completely smooth.

2. Add the remaining base ingredients together with 1 cup of water and blend well.

3. Add one of the flavorings and pulse-blend a few times, to give you more of a chunky soup.

JUICE COMBINATIONS

While you can experiment with juicing of any combination of vegetables and fruits, here are a few suggestions of proven and delicious combinations for inexperienced juicers:

→ Spinach, green apple, and cucumber

→ Spinach, green apple, celery, and lime

→ Spinach, romaine, celery, cucumber, and mint

→ Spinach, kale, cilantro, and lemon

→ Beet, carrot, apple, and ginger

→ Beet, strawberry, and romaine lettuce

→ Dandelion, cabbage, and celery

→ Grapefruit, spinach, apple, and ginger

→ Orange, pineapple, carrot, and lime

→ Carrot, celery, tomato, and lime

If your juice doesn't taste sweet enough, add apples and carrots. If it's too strong, you can remove ginger or lime. For increased anti-inflammatory properties, add a small piece of turmeric root (about one inch) to any juice.

Try to make your own juice combinations by choosing and juicing together:

→ 1 sweet fruit or vegetable (apples, carrots, beets, fennel)

→ 2–3 neutral vegetables (zucchini, cucumber, winter squash, lettuce/spinach) that will make the base of your juice

→ A small amount from the strong flavor category (ginger, lemon/lime, dark leafy greens, celery)

RAW JAM BLUEPRINT

It is really simple to make your own jam from fresh fruits. It's much healthier and tastes so much fresher than the sugar-laden conventional jam. Blend berries or fruits, sweetener and a thickener. Easy!

INGREDIENTS

2 cups fruit (strawberries, raspberries, blackberries, blueberries, figs, oranges, apricots or other fruit you like)
2 tbsp chia seeds ground to powder
1-2 tbsp maple syrup or ½ cup of soaked pitted dates
1 tbsp lemon juice
1 tbsp lemon zest (optional)
4 tbsp water (more or less according to the consistency of your jam)

DIRECTIONS

1. Place soaked (30–60 minutes, or until soft) and pitted dates or sweetener, with water in a high-speed blender and blend to break up dates. Add more water if necessary.

2. Place chia seeds and half of the fruit into the blender on low speed, pulse-blend a few times.

3. Add the remaining fruit and pulse-blend a few times on low speed to create a chunky texture.

4. Pour the mixture into a mason jar or another container, add lemon juice, and stir with a spoon until it is blended.

5. Taste for sweetness. Add more sweetener if needed.

6. Refrigerate in an airtight jar for 30 minutes, until the jam becomes firm.

NON-DAIRY MILK OR YOGURT

Delicious non-dairy milks can be made from

- → Nuts: almonds, cashews, Brazil nuts, walnuts, pecans, or coconut

- → Seeds: hemp, sunflower, flax, or pumpkin

- → Grains: rice, oats, quinoa, buckwheat, barley, or rye

To create a non-dairy cultured beverage or yogurt, add a tiny amount of lemon juice to your final product.

INGREDIENTS

1 cup soaked nuts, seeds, or grains
3 cups water
Sweetener (optional): 2 dates, maple syrup, agave, coconut nectar, blackstrap molasses, coconut sugar, Stevia, honey, Xylitol
Flavorings (optional): ½ tsp vanilla, cinnamon, cocoa, nutmeg, ginger, cloves, pumpkin pie spice

DIRECTIONS

1. Soak nuts or grains for 8–12 hours.

2. Nuts: drain, rinse, and put them in a high-speed blender.

3. Grains: drain, rinse, and cook or sprout before adding them in a blender. Sprouting will preserve more nutrients.

4. Add 3 cups of water to the blender. If you want your milk thicker, add less; if you want it thinner, add more. For a cream, add only 1–2 cups.

5. Blend until smooth. High performance blenders will do an amazing job, but other blenders are functional as well.

6. Some nuts (such as almonds or coconut) or grains will create a grainy consistency that you need to strain through a strainer or a cloth. Save the

pulp for baking or to use in other dishes. Other nuts such as cashews create a super creamy consistency without the need for straining.

7. Optional: Put the milk back into the blender with sweeteners and flavorings of your choice and blend well.

The milks can be stored in the refrigerator for several days. Use them for super creamy and delicious smoothies, or in combination with frozen bananas or mangoes for a delicious plant-based ice cream.

NON-DAIRY MAYONNAISE

Use mayonnaise for sandwiches, wraps, salads, and dressings. For 1 cup of mayonnaise, use following:

INGREDIENTS

1 cup cashews (soaked for 4 hours)
½ cup extra-virgin olive oil
½ tbsp sweetener of your choice
2 tbsp lemon juice
½ tbsp apple cider vinegar
¼ tsp dry mustard
Pinch of salt

DIRECTIONS

1. Place everything except oil into a high-powered blender and blend until very smooth.

2. Then start slowly pouring in olive oil while blending until it is creamy.

3. Taste and adjust seasonings accordingly.

4. The mixture thickens in the refrigerator as it cools down. If you don't eat it immediately (it's that good), it will last one week.

FLAX-EGGS FOR BAKING

Great substitute for eggs in baking are so called flax-eggs, made easily from ground flax seeds and water. The following recipe makes six flax-eggs.

DIRECTIONS

1. Grind 1/3 cup of flax seeds in the blender until they become powder.

2. Slowly add 1 cup of water until the texture becomes gooey.

3. Three tablespoons of this mixture yields one "egg."

4. Keep your flax-eggs in the refrigerator up to six days.

I have used these flax-eggs for baking and to make potato cakes (latkes), or other veggie patties and burgers that call for eggs in the recipe.

PROTEIN COOKIES AND ENERGY BARS BLUEPRINT

These are extremely easy to make and are so much more nutritious than the commercial versions. They are completely customizable to your liking since you have control over all the ingredients.

Choose one ingredient from each group and get creative. If your dough is too dry, add more liquid. If it is too runny, add more dry ingredients until it has a spreadable consistency. The more often you make your cookies, the more proficient you will get and your creations will be delicious.

This recipe makes about 16 cookies/bars, 2 oz and 200 calories each. The nutritional values and calories will vary slightly depending on your ingredients. It takes about 15 minutes to make the dough, and another 15 minutes to bake (or chill if you make them raw).

INGREDIENTS

Dry base: 1 cup
Combine two or more of the following: brown rice flour, whole wheat flour, buckwheat flour, garbanzo bean flour, quinoa flour, spelt flour, cocoa, or protein powder from hemp, brown rice, sunflower, pumpkin, or peas.

Wet base: 16-once can or 1 ½ cups cooked
White, black, pinto, adzuki, or garbanzo beans (drained)

Fluffy ingredient: 1 ½ cups
Puffed quinoa, puffed rice, puffed millet, or oats

Sticky ingredient: ½ cup
Peanut butter, almond butter, cashew butter, coconut manna, pureed pumpkin, mashed avocado, flax seed paste (¼ cup ground mixed with ¼ cup of water)

Soft sweet fruit: ¼ cup
Chopped pitted dates, applesauce, mashed banana, mashed pineapple, raw figs, soaked raisins or figs

Sweetener: ¼ cup
Maple syrup, agave syrup, coconut nectar, honey, brown rice syrup, barley syrup, Stevia

Flavoring: 1 cup
Raisins, dried cranberries, dried mulberries, dried apricots, dried cherries, dried blueberries, dried bananas chips, chopped nuts, poppy seeds, chocolate chips, cacao nibs, coconut flakes, dried cereal

Dry spice (optional): 1 tsp
Cinnamon, nutmeg, cardamom, ginger, instant coffee, instant green tea

Extract (optional): 1 tsp
Lemon, almond, coconut, vanilla, coffee

Salty flavor (optional): ¼ tsp
Sea salt

DIRECTIONS

1. Place one ingredient from each group (except the crunchy flavorings) into a high-powered blender or food processor and mix well. You may need to pulse-blend if you are using a blender.

2. If the dough is too dry, add more water, if it is too runny, add more dry ingredients. It should be the consistency of conventional cookie dough.

3. Blend in the crunchy flavorings gently. Don't over-process—you want to taste the pieces.

4. Use a silicone baking pan, or a pan greased with coconut oil or covered with parchment paper.

5. For bars, pour the dough into the pan and push it around so it is evenly thick.

6. For cookies, make balls and flatten them on the baking pan.

7. Bake at 350 degrees for 15–20 minutes.

Store your cookies in an airtight container (a mason jar works great). Refrigeration is not necessary, but storing them in the fridge will extend their shelf life. This may not be necessary though, because you may finish them before you have a chance to store them. I always have problems with self-discipline when I have many of these yummy cookies around. For these problems, a great solution is to freeze them, and pull out only a few each day.

The cost is about $10 per batch, which is around $0.40 per bar/cookie. This is much cheaper than commercially made bars and cookies, which can easily go over $2 per piece. Not to mention that yours are much healthier, fresher, and made with love.

RAW PROTEIN COOKIES AND ENERGY BARS

You can easily transform the above creations into raw bars and cookies. Make them moist and chewy (just form the dough and chill) or crunchy (put them in a dehydrator for a few hours). To make delicious raw bars:

1. Eliminate canned or cooked beans. Use sprouted beans instead, or none.

2. Eliminate the dry flours and use less dry ingredients, or use almond or cashew meal instead. You can make your own meal from the nuts in the power-blender.

3. You may need to increase the sticky ingredients and sweeteners by fifty percent.

EXAMPLE: QUICK AND EASY RAW PROTEIN BAR

This is a raw protein bar, made from the blueprint above. The preparation time is about 15 minutes, and freezing time is 15 minutes. It is a quick, easy, and very delightful snack. Who says that baking is difficult and baked goods are not healthy?

INGREDIENTS

½ cup unsweetened vegan protein powder (dry base)
½ cup almond meal (dry base)
1 cup oats blended into a flour (fluffy ingredient)
½ cup rice crisp cereal (fluffy ingredient)
½ cup natural peanut butter, almond butter, or sunflower seed butter (sticky ingredient)
½ cup pure maple syrup (or liquid sweetener of choice) (sweetener)
½ cup mini dark chocolate chips or cacao nibs (flavorings)
½ cup raisins (flavorings)
1 tsp pure vanilla extract (Extract, optional)
¼ tsp sea salt (optional)

DIRECTIONS

1. Mix the oat flour, protein powder, rice crisp, and salt together in a large bowl or a food processor.

2. Add in the nut/seed butter, maple syrup, chocolate chips, and vanilla. Stir well to combine. If the mixture is a bit dry, add a splash of liquid (water or non-dairy milk) and mix again.

3. Line an 8-inch square pan with a piece of parchment paper or use silicone forms.

4. Press the dough into the pan and push with hands or roll out with a pastry roller until smooth.

5. Set into the freezer for 15 minutes.

6. Remove from the freezer and slice into bars.

EXAMPLE: RAW BANANA NUT BAR

INGREDIENTS

1 cup raw protein powder (vanilla flavor, if you wish) (dry base)
½ cup raw coconut flour
2 cups mashed banana (wet base, soft fruit)
1 cup raw sliced almonds or nut of choice (flavorings)
¼ cup raw coconut sugar or desired sweetener (sweetener, optional)
1 tsp vanilla extract
1 tsp cinnamon
4 tbsp water (optional)

DIRECTIONS

1. Place all ingredients in a bowl or food processor and mix until smooth.

2. Place the dough in a pan lined with parchment paper, or use a silicone pan. Push or roll out the dough until even and smooth.

3. Put into the freezer for 15 minutes.

4. Slice into 16 bars.

5. Keep refrigerated to keep the bars firm.

EXAMPLE: RAW LOW-CARB PROTEIN NUT COOKIE

INGREDIENTS

1 cup protein powder
1 cup almond flour
½ cup cashew or peanut butter
¼ cup cashews
¼ cup sunflower seeds
¼ cup pumpkin seeds
¼ cup hemp seeds
¼ cup agave syrup

DIRECTIONS

1. Place all ingredients in a bowl or food processor and mix until smooth.

2. Roll into 1-inch balls, then flatten thin and put on a dehydrator sheet.

3. Dehydrate for one to two days on 105 F until you achieve desired dryness and crunchiness.

RAW CONFECTIONS BLUEPRINT

Your imagination is the only limiting factor in the variety of confections that you can create. Keep experimenting and try combining different soaked dried fruits with fresh fruits, nuts, and seeds.

Use chopped raisins, dates, or figs, and combine them with ground or chopped nuts, ground or whole seeds, and mashed fresh fruits. If you desire a chocolate taste, add raw cacao or powdered carob. For easy handling, roll your final confections in shredded or ground coconut. Chill to get firm.

EXAMPLE: SIMPLE COCONUT BALLS DELIGHT

This is one of the simplest desserts to make and because of that, it is my favorite.

INGREDIENTS

2 cups almonds (or other nuts or nut meal)
1 ½ cups raisins
1 cup dried shredded coconut

DIRECTIONS

Blend nuts and raisins in a blender or food processor until you get a dough-like consistency. If you use almond or cashew meal, you can blend everything by hand in a bowl. Mold the dough into balls and roll them in coconut. Refrigerate or freeze for one hour or until they are firm.

SIMPLE CABBAGE DELIGHT

This is my favorite meal. It is easy to prepare and is low in calories. It's great for those evenings when you still feel hungry but you should not be eating too many more calories.

DIRECTIONS

1. In a high-powered blender, shred or pulse-blend one head of white cabbage.

2. Add sea salt, black pepper, a tiny bit of sweetener of your choice (I use Stevia), and lemon juice from one or more lemons. Be creative, please your taste buds.

3. Optional: add almonds, flax seeds, coconut, or shredded carrot to make your cabbage taste slightly different each time.

4. Blend well and let it set for 5–10 minutes before eating.

PLAY WITH YOUR FOOD

All of these recipes are very simple to make and they should encourage you to play with your food. They will stimulate your creativity as well as your appetite. You will soon discover how delicious the plant-based meals can taste, and how simple they are to make. Remember to use your seasonings just to complement, not to replace, the natural flavors of plants. The less you cook and the more raw ingredients you use, the simpler your cooking life will get.

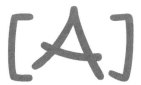

ACKNOWLEDGMENTS

This book has been in the process of creation for a long time. At first, it was only my personal research for my personal health benefits, which turned out to be so impressive that I had to let everybody know through the creation of this work. I am truly thankful to all the great researchers and professionals whose works I have been studying. Thank you Dr. Campbell, Dr. Esselstyn, Dr. McDougall, Dr. Ornish, Dr. Barnard, Dr. Greger, Jeff Novick, Ann Wigmore, and many more, who helped me to realize the amazing benefits of eating plants and for becoming who I am now.

A huge thanks to my mom, who lives over 6,000 miles away and who has been my biggest supporter and the perfect "experiment rabbit." She faithfully followed my every step and was doing everything I was doing, starting from vegetarian, then fully plant-based, and finally raw. It takes a lot of courage and humility for a mother to let herself be guided by her daughter. Thank you, Mom, you are my idol!

Many thanks go to all my fitness students, friends, and tennis partners, who were patient with me as I constantly ranted about the new information and knowledge that I was acquiring. Those who adopted the plant-based lifestyle have helped me to realize all the possible issues and difficulties that people can have during the transition to a plant-based lifestyle. Thank you for being brave and joining me on this journey.

Lastly, this book would sound like a Czech-Swedish-American concoction if my girls—editors and proofreaders—Janet Kolbu, Doree Gerold, and Wendy Brynford-Jones, didn't help me eliminate my "accent" from the pages. Thank you, girls, for making me sound like an American, and thanks to Maria Rosetti for the lovely cover art.

Thanks to all the organic farmers in the world, your hard work is truly appreciated. Finally, thank You, dear reader, for reading my work.

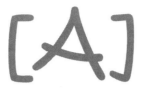

ABOUT THE AUTHOR

Suzanna McGee is a former Ms. Natural Olympia drug-free bodybuilding champion, now competitive tennis player and expert athletic trainer, certified by the National Academy of Sports Medicine as a performance enhancement specialist and corrective exercise specialist. She has over twenty years of experience in athletic training.

With great success, Suzanna has become a plant-based athlete and has earned a certificate in plant-based nutrition at eCornell University. This added focus on plant-based nutrition completes the maximum health and performance package from which every athlete and non-athlete will benefit.

Suzanna is the author of *Tennis Fitness for the Love of it: a Mindful Approach to Fitness for Injury-Free Tennis* and *Racquetball and Squash: Conditioning and Injury Prevention*, two popular books on recreating balance in the body to prevent overuse injuries in athletes.

With her teaching and writings, Suzanna possesses the tremendous ability to inspire athletes to be the best that they can be. Suzanna's special training style, which combines many different techniques of training, healing, and injury prevention, brings a lot of success and great results to anybody who learns to master it.

Besides her love of sports, learning, and teaching, Suzanna has two master's degrees in computer science, and speaks six languages. This Czech native resides with her chocolate Labrador in Venice Beach, California.

You can reach Suzanna via her website at www.TennisFitnessLove.com or email at suzanna@TennisFitnessLove.com.

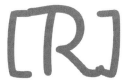

RESOURCES

To further open your horizons and learn more about whole foods plant-based nutrition, performance training, and health and longevity, here are a few resources listed. The list is far from complete, but it is a good start.

BOOKS

The China Study, Colin Campbell, Ph.D.

Whole, Colin Campbell, Ph.D.

Prevent and Reverse Heart Disease, Caldwell Esselstyn, M.D.

Becoming Vegan, Brenda Davis, RD

The Starch Solution, John McDougall, M.D.

Eat to Live, Joel Fuhrman, M.D.

The Pleasure Trap, Doug Lisle, Ph.D.

The Food Revolution, John Robbins

Thrive, Brendan Brazier

Green for Life, Victoria Boutenko

12 Steps to Raw Foods: How to End Your Dependency on Cooked Food, Victoria Boutenko

The World Peace Diet, Will Tuttle, Ph.D.

21-Day Weight Loss Kickstart, Neal Barnard, M.D.

The Engine 2 Diet, Rip Esselstyn

Comfortably Unaware, Richard Oppenlander, Ph.D.

Timeless Secrets of Health and Rejuvenation, Andreas Moritz

Food for Nation, Eric Schlosser

Overdosed America, John Abramson, M.D.

COOKBOOKS

Everyday Happy Herbivore, Lindsey S. Nixon

The China Study Cookbook, LeAnn Campbell

Forks Over Knives - The Cookbook, Del Sroufe

Recipes for Longer Life, Ann Wigmore

The McDougall Quick and Easy Cookbook, John McDougall, M.D. and Mary McDougall

Appetite for Reduction: 125 Fast and Filling Low-Fat Vegan Recipes, Isa Chandra Moskowitz

The Get Healthy, Go Vegan Cookbook, Neal Barnard, M.D.

Juicing With The Omega Juicer, Annie Deeter

Live Raw Around The World, Mimi Kirk

Raw Food Made Easy for 1 or 2 people, Jennifer Cornbleet

MOVIES AND DOCUMENTARIES

Forks Over Knives

The Gerson Miracle

Fat, Sick, and Nearly Dead

Food, INC

Vegucated

Fresh

Earthlings

Processed People

EDUCATION

eCornell certificate in Plant Based Nutrition:
www.ecornell.com/certificates/plant-based-nutrition

The World Peace Diet Facilitator Training Program:
www.worldpeacemastery.com

The McDougall Nutrition Programs:
www.drmcdougall.com/health/programs

Farms 2 Forks Weekend Immersions:
www.farms2forks.com

The Hippocrates Health Educator Program:
www.hippocratesinst.org/health-educator-program

WEBSITES

www.doctorklaper.com	Dr. Michael Klaper
www.drfuhrman.com	Dr. Joel Fuhrman
www.drmcdougall.com	Dr. John McDougall

www.heartattackproof.com	Dr. Caldwell B. Esselstyn
www.jeffnovick.com	Jeff Novick, RD
www.nutritionfacts.org	Dr. Michael Greger
www.pcrm.org	Physicians committee for responsible medicine
www.thechinastudy.com	Colin Campbell, Ph.D.
www.worldpeacediet.org	Will Tuttle, Ph.D.

www.growingyourgreens.com	Advice on growing your own food in urban areas
www.happycow.net	All about vegan, worldwide: restaurant and store locator, recipes, products, articles
www.okraw.com	Video advice on eating a raw plant-based diet
www.sproutpeople.org	Sprouting advice, seeds and tools
www.vegancuts.com	Deals on vegan food, body care, fashion and other
www.vegnews.com	Vegan lifestyle magazine
www.vegsource.com	Vegetarian and vegan information

www.vitamix.com	Power blenders (the Ferraris of blenders)
www.blendtec.com	
www.nutribullet.com	Small travel blender
www.omegajuicers.com	Quality juicers

www.edenfoods.com	Non-GMO grains and beans, in BPA-free cans
www.manitobaharvest.com	High quality, chemical-free hemp food products
www.montanaglutenfree.com	Raw and gluten-free grains and flours
www.nuts.com	Nuts, grains, dried fruits
www.znaturalfoods.com	Raw, organic foods and super-foods at great prices

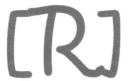

REFERENCES

American College of Sports Medicine, American Dietetic Association, and Dietitians of Canada. Position stand: Nutrition and athletic performance. Med. Sci. Sports Exerc. 32(12):2130–2145. 2000.

American College of Sports Medicine. Position stand: Exercise and fluid replacement. Med. Sci. Sports Exerc. 28:2130–2145. 1996.

American Dietetic Association; Dietitians of Canada; American College of Sports Medicine, Rodriguez NR, Di Marco NM, Langley S. American College of Sports Medicine position stand. Nutrition and athletic performance. Med Sci Sports Exerc. 2009 Mar;41(3):709-31.

Appleby P, Roddam A, Allen N, Key T. Comparative fracture risk in vegetarians and nonvegetarians in EPIC-Oxford. Eur J Clin Nutr 2007;61:1400–6.

Appleby PN, Davey GK, Key TJ. Hypertension and blood pressure among meat eaters, fish eaters, vegetarians and vegans in EPIC-Oxford. Public Health Nutrition 2002;5:645-654.

Armstrong BK. Absorption of vitamin B12 from the human colon. Am J Clin Nutr 1968; 21:298-9.

Balshaw TG, Bampouras TM, Barry TJ, Sparks SA. The effect of acute taurine ingestion on 3-km running performance in trained middle-distance runners. Amino Acids.2013 Feb;44(2):555-61.

Barnard ND, Cohen J, Jenkins DJA, et al. A low-fat vegan diet and a conventional diabetes diet in the treatment of type-2 diabetes: a randomized, controlled, 74-wk clinical trial. Am J Clin Nutr 2009;89(suppl):1588S–96S.

Barnard ND, Cohen J, Jenkins DJA, et al. A low-fat vegan diet improves glycemic control and cardiovascular risk factors in a randomized clinical trial in individuals with type 2 diabetes. Diabetes Care 2006;29:1777–83.

Barr SI, Rideout CA. Nutritional considerations for vegetarian athletes. Nutrition. 2004; 20(7Y8):696Y703.

Barzel US, Massey LK. Excess dietary protein can adversely affect bone. Journal of Nutrition, 1998, 128:1051–1053.

Bazzano LA, Serdula MK, Liu S. Dietary intake of fruits and vegetables and risk of cardiovascular disease. Curr Atheroscler Rep 2003;5:492–9.

Beyranvand, M., Khalafi, M., et al. Effect of Taurine Supplementation on Exercise Capacity of Patients with Heart Failure. Journal of Cardiology. May 2011. 57(3), 333-335.

Birdsall TC. Therapeutic applications of taurine. Altern Med Rev. 1998 Apr;3(2):128-36.

Botterill, C., and C. Wilson. Overtraining: Emotional and interdisciplinary dimensions. In: Enhancing Recovery: Preventing Underperformance in Athletes. M. Kellman, ed. Champaign, IL: Human Kinetics, 2002. pp. 143–160.

Brathwaite N, Fraser HS, Modeste N, Broome H, King R. Obesity, diabetes, hypertension, and vegetarian status among Seventh-day Adventists in Barbados: preliminary results. Ethn Dis 2003;13:34–9.

Callender ST, Spray GH. Latent pernicious anemia. Br J Haematol 1962;8:230-240.

Campbell B, Kreider RB, Ziegenfuss T, et al. International Society of Sports Nutrition position stand: protein and exercise. J. Int. Soc. Sports. Nutr. 2007; 4:8.

Campbell, T. C. & Campbell, T. M., II. The China Study, Startling Implications for Diet, Weight Loss, and Long-Term Health. (BenBella Books, Inc., 2005).

Carlsen MH, Halvorsen BL, Holte K, et al. The total antioxidant content of more than 3100 foods, beverages, spices, herbs and supplements used worldwide. Nutrition J. 2010; 9(3):1475Y2891.

Carroll, K. K. in Animal and Vegetable Proteins in Lipid Metabolism and Atherosclerosis (eds M.J. Gibney & D. Kritchevsky) 9-17 (Alan R. Liss, Inc., 1983).

Chen HI. Effects of 30-h sleep loss on cardiorespiratory functions at rest and in exercise. Med Sci Sports Exerc. 1991 Feb;23(2):193-8.

Chiu JF, Lan SJ, Yang CY, et al. Long-term vegetarian diet and bone mineral density in postmenopausal Taiwanese women. Calcif Tissue Int 1997;60:245–9.

Craig WJ. Health effects of vegan diets. Am J Clin Nutr. 2009 May;89(5):1627S-1633S.

Craig WJ. Iron status of vegetarians. Am J Clin Nutr 1994;59(suppl):1233S–7S.

Craig WJ. Nutrition concerns and health effects of vegetarian diets. Nutr Clin Pract. 2010 Dec;25(6):613-20.

Craig WJ, Mangels AR. American Dietetic Association. Position of the American Dietetic Association: vegetarian diets. J. Am. Diet. Assoc. 2009; 109(7):1266Y82.

Cuisinier C, Ward RJ, Francaux M, et al. Changes in plasma and urinary taurine and amino acids in runners immediately and 24h after a marathon. Amino Acids. 2001; 20(1):13Y23.

Davey GK, Spencer EA, Appleby PN, Allen NE, Knox KH, Key TJ. EPIC-Oxford: lifestyle characteristics and nutrient intakes in a cohort of 33,883 meat-eaters and 31,546 non meat-eaters in the UK. Public Health Nutr 2003;6:259–69.

Davis B, Melina V. Becoming Vegan: Summertown, TN: Book Publishing Co; 2000.

Dawson R, Jr., Biasetti M, Messina S, Dominy J. The cytoprotective role of taurine in exercise-induced muscle injury. Amino Acids.2002 Jun;22(4):309-24.

De Biase SG, Fernandes SF, Gianini RJ, Duarte JL. Vegetarian diet and cholesterol and triglyceride levels. Arq Bras Cardiol 2007;88:35–9.

Deutz RC, Benardot D, Martin DE, Cody MM. Relationship between energy deficits and body composition in elite female gymnasts and runners. Med Sci Sports Exerc. 2000 Mar;32(3):659-68.

Dewell A, Weidner G, Sumner MD, Chi CS, Ornish D. A very-low fat vegan diet increases intake of protective dietary factors and decreases intake of pathogenic dietary factors. J Am Diet Assoc 2008;108:347–56.

Dietary Reference Intakes for Energy, Carbohydrate, Fiber, Fat,Fatty Acids, Cholesterol, Protein, and Amino Acids (Macronutrients)National Academy of Sciences. 2005.

Dietary Reference Intakes for Energy, Carbohydrates, Fiber, Fat, Protein and Amino Acids (Macronutrients). Food and Nutrition Board, Institute of Medicine. Washington, DC: National Academies Press; 2002.

Dietary Reference Intakes, Food and Drug Administration. (The recommendations for protein are 56g/day for adult males and 46 g/day for adult females. The suggested caloric intake is 2301-3720 for a 5'11" man and 1816-2807 for a 5'5" woman. At 4 calories of protein per gram, this works out to 8.0-12.3% protein for men and 6.6-10.1%)

Djoussé L, Arnett DK, Coon H, Province MA, Moore LL, Ellison RC. Fruit and vegetable consumption and LDL cholesterol: the National Heart, Lung, and Blood Institute Family Heart Study. Am J Clin Nutr 2004;79:213–7.

Doi T, Matsuo T, Sugawara M, Matsumoto K, Minehira K, Hamada K, Okamura K, Suzuki M. New approach for weight reduction by a combination of diet, light resistance exercise and the timing of ingesting a protein supplement. Asia Pacific journal of clinical nutrition. 2001;10(3):226-32.

Elkan AC, Sjöberg B, Kolsrud B, Ringertz B, Hafström I, Frostegård J. Gluten-free vegan diet induces decreased LDL and oxidized LDL levels and raised atheroprotective natural antibodies against phosphorylcholine in patients with rheumatoid arthritis: a randomized study. Arthritis Res Ther. 2008;10(2):R34.

Elmadfa I, Singer I. Vitamin B-12 and homocysteine status among vegetarians: a global perspective. Am J Clin Nutr 2009;89(suppl):1693S–8S.

Esselstyn CB Jr. Updating a 12-year experience with arrest and reversal therapy for coronary heart disease (an overdue requiem for palliative cardiology). Am J Cardiol. 1999 Aug 1;84(3):339-41, A8.

Esselstyn, C. B., Ellis, S. G., Medendorp, S. V. & Crowe, T. D. A strategy to arrest and reverse coronary artery disease: a 5-year longitudinal study of a single physician's practice. J. Family Practice 41, 560-568 (1995).

Exercise and Fluid Replacement Position Stand, American College of Sports Medicine, Med Sci Sports Exer. 2007:39;377-390.

Faigenbaum, A.D., P. Mediate, and D. Rota. Sleep need in high school athletes. Strength Cond. J. 24(4):18–19.2002.

Food and Nutrition Board, "Dietary Reference Intakes for Energy, Carbohydrates, Fiber, Fat, Protein and Amino Acids (Macronutrients)," National Academy of Sciences (2002): 10-1.

Food and Nutrition Board, Institute of Medicine. Vitamin B12: Dietary Reference Intakes for thiamin, riboflavin, niacin, vitamin B6, folate, vitamin B12, pantothenic acid. Washington, DC: Biotin, and Choline. National Academy Press, 1998;306–56.

Fraser G. Risk factors and disease among vegans. In: Fraser G ed. Diet, life expectancy, and chronic disease. Studies of Seventh-day Adventists and other vegetarians. New York, NY: Oxford University Press, 2003:231–9.

Fraser GE. Vegetarian diets: what do we know of their effects on common chronic diseases? Am J Clin Nutr 2009;89(suppl):1607S–12S.

Fuhrman J, Ferreri DM. Fueling the vegetarian (vegan) athlete. Curr Sports Med Rep. 2010 Jul-Aug;9(4):233-41.

Garcia AL, Koebnick C, Dagnelie PC, Strassner C, Elmadfa I, Katz N, Leitzmann C, Hoffmann I. Long-term strict raw food diet is associated with favourable plasma beta-carotene and low plasma lycopene concentrations in Germans. Br J Nutr. 2008 Jun;99(6):1293-300.

Galloway SDR, Talanian JL, Shoveller AK, et al. Seven days of oral taurine supplementation does not increase muscle taurine content or alter substrate metabolism during prolonged exercise in humans. J. Appl. Physiol. 2008; 105:643Y51.

George D F, Bilek M M, and McKenzie D R. Non-thermal effects in the microwave induced unfolding of proteins observed by chaperone binding.

Gertjan Schaafsma, "The Protein Digestiblity-Corrected Amino Acid Score," Journal of Nutrition 130 (2000):1865S-1867S.

Gibson RS. Content and bioavailability of trace elements in vegetarian diets. Am J Clin Nutr 1994;59(suppl):1223S–32S.

Gleeson M. Can nutrition limit exercise-induced immunodepression? Nutr. Rev. 2006; 64(3):119Y31.

Goodman CA, Horvath D, Stathis C, et al. Taurine supplementation increases skeletal muscle force production and protects muscle function during and after high-frequency in vitro stimulation.J Appl Physiol. 2009 Jul;107(1):144-54.

Haddad EH, Berk LS, Kettering JD, Hubbard RW, Peters WR. Dietary intake and biochemical, hematologic, and immune status of vegans compared with nonvegetarians. Am J Clin Nutr 1999;70(suppl):586S–93S.

Halbesma N, Bakker SJ, Jansen DF, et al. High protein intake associates with cardiovascular events but not with loss of renal function. J. Am. Soc. Nephrol. 2009; 20(8):1797Y804.

Hallert C, Grännö C, Grant C, Hultén S, Midhagen G, Ström M, Svensson H, Valdimarsson T, Wickström T. Quality of life of adult coeliac patients treated for 10 years. Scand J Gastroenterol. 1998 Sep;33(9):933-8.

Hamilton B. Vitamin D and human skeletal muscle. Scand. J. Med. Sci. Sports. 2010; 20(2):182Y90.

Hamilton, E., Berg, HJ., et al. The Effect of Taurine Depletion on the Contractile Properties and Fatigue in Fast-Twitch Skeletal Muscle of the Mouse. Amino acids. October 2001. 31(3), 273-280.

Hawley, John. Optimizing Muscle Mass Through Exercise and Nutrient Availability. International Conference on Strength Training. Norway: Oslo.2012.

Heaney RP. Protein and calcium: antagonists or synergists? American Journal of Clinical Nutrition, 2002, 75:609–610.

Hemmings, B., M. Smith, J. Graydon, and R. Dyson. Effects of massage on physiological restoration, perceived recovery, and repeated sports performance. Br. J. Sports Med. 34(2):109–114. 2000.

Herbert V. Vitamin B12: Plant sources, requirements, and assay. Am J Clin Nutr 1988;48:852-858.

Herrman W, Obeid R. Causes and early diagnosis of vitamin B12 deficiency. Dtsch. Arztebl. Int. 2008; 105(40):680Y5.

Holick MF. Sunlight, UV-radiation, vitamin D and skin cancer: how much sunlight do we need? Adv Exp Med Biol 2008;624:1–15.

Holmstrup, M., et al. Effect of Meal Frequency on Glucose and Insulin Excursions Over the Course of a Day. European E-Journal of Clinical Nutrition and Metabolism. 2010. 5(6), e277-2280.

Hu FB et al. Dietary protein and risk of ischemic heart disease in women. American Journal of Clinical Nutrition, 1999, 70:221–227.

Hudson-Walters, P. Sleep, the athlete and performance. Strength Cond. J. 24(2):17–24. 2004.

Hunt JR. Bioavailability of iron, zinc, and other trace minerals from vegetarian diets. Am. J. Clin. Nutr. 2003; 78(Suppl.):633SY9S.

Hunt JR. Moving towards a plant-based diet: are iron and zinc at risk? Nutr Rev 2002;60:127–34.

Imagawa TF, Hirano I, Utsuki K, et al. Caffeine and taurine enhance endurance performance. Int J Sports Med. 2009 Jul;30(7):485-8.

Institute of Medicine, Food and Nutrition Board: Dietary Reference Intakes for Thiamin, Riboflavin, Niacin, Vitamin B-6, Folate, Vitamin B-12, Pantothenic Acid, Biotin, and Choline. Washington, DC: National Academy Press, 1998.

Institute of Medicine. Dietary Reference Intakes for Water, Potassium, Sodium, Chloride and Sulfate. Washington, DC: National Academies Press, 2004.

Jacobs DR Jr., Haddad EH, Lanou AJ, Messina MJ. Food, plant food, and vegetarian diets in the US dietary guidelines: conclusions of an expert panel. Am J Clin Nutr 2009;89(suppl):1549S–52S.

Jacobsen MF. Six arguments for a greener diet: how a more plant-based diet could save your health and the environment. Washington, DC: Center for Science in the Public Interest, 2006.

Janelle KC, Barr SI. Nutrient intakes and eating behavior scores of vegetarian and nonvegetarian women. J Am Diet Assoc. 1995 Feb;95(2):180-6.

Kelly JH Jr., Sabate J. Nuts and coronary heart disease: an epidemiological perspective. Br J Nutr 2006;96(suppl):S61–7.

Kendler BS. Taurine: an overview of its role in preventive medicine. Prev Med. 1989 Jan;18(1):79-100.

Kentta, G., and P. Hassmen. Underrecovery and overtraining: A conceptual model. In: Enhancing Recovery: Preventing Underperformance in Athletes. M. Kellman, ed. Champaign, IL: Human Kinetics, 2002. pp. 57–77.

Key TJ, Appleby PN, Rosell MS. Health effects of vegetarian and vegan diets. Proc Nutr Soc 2006;65:35–41

Key TJ, Fraser GE, Thorogood M, et al. Mortality in vegetarians and nonvegetarians: detailed findings from a collaborative analysis of 5 prospective studies. Am J Clin Nutr 1999;70(suppl):516S–24S.

Kreider RB, Campbell B. Protein for exercise and recovery. Phys. Sportsmed. 2009; 37(2):13Y21.

Kubbitz, K.A., D.M. Landers, S.J. Petruzzelo, and J. Han. The effects of acute and chronic exercise on sleep. A meta-analytical review. Sports Med. 21:277–291. 1996.

Kurtzweil , Paula. "'Daily Values' Encourage Healthy Diet," U.S. Food and Drug Administration, 2003.

Laidlaw SA, Grosvenor M, Kopple JD (1990). The taurine content of common foodstuffs.JPEN J Parenter Enteral Nutr. 1990 Mar-Apr;14(2):183-8.

Laidlaw SA, Shultz TD, Cecchino JT, Kopple JD. Plasma and urine taurine levels in vegans. Am J Clin Nutr. 1988 Apr;47(4):660-3.

Lambert CP, Flynn MG. Fatigue during high-intensity intermittent exercise: application to bodybuilding. Sports Med. 2002;32(8):511-22.

Lamprecht M, Hofmann P, Greilberger JF, Schwaberger G. Increased lipid peroxidation in trained men after 2 weeks of antioxidant supplementation. Int. J. Sport. Nutr. Exerc. Metab. 2009; 19(4):385Y99.

Larson E. Vegetarian diet for exercise and athletic training and performing: an update. Vegetarian Nutrition. Vegetarian Dietetic Practice Group of the American Dietetic Association. http://www.andrews.edu/NUFS/vegathletes.htm Accessed November 5, 2002.

Larsson CL, Johansson GK. Dietary intake and nutritional status of young vegans and omnivores in Sweden. Am J Clin Nutr 2002;76:100–6.

Larsson CL, Johansson GK. Young Swedish vegans have different sources of nutrients than young omnivores. J Am Diet Assoc 2005;105:1438–41.

Larsson, S. C. & Orsini, N. Red meat and processed meat consumption and all-cause mortality: a meta-analysis. Am. J. Epidemiol. 179, 282-289 (2013).

Lau EMC, Kwok T, Woo J, Ho SC. Bone mineral density in Chinese elderly female vegetarians, vegans, lacto-ovegetarians and omnivores. Eur J Clin Nutr 1998;52:60–4.

Leitzmann C. Vegetarian diets: what are the advantages? Forum Nutr. 2005;(57):147-56.

Lemon PW, Tarnopolsky MA, MacDougall JD, Atkinson SA. Protein requirements and muscle mass/strength changes during intensive training in novice bodybuilders. J Appl Physiol. 1992 Aug;73(2):767-75.

Lemon PW, Tarnopolsky MA, MacDougall JD, Atkinson SA. Protein requirements and muscle mass/strength changes during intensive training in novice bodybuilders. J Appl Physiol. 1992 Aug;73(2):767-75.

Lemon PW. Effects of exercise on dietary protein requirements. Int J Sport Nutr. 1998 Dec;8(4):426-47.

Liu RH. Health benefits of fruits and vegetables are from additive and synergistic combinations of phytochemicals. Am J Clin Nutr 2003;78(suppl):517S–20S.

Liu RH. Potential synergy of phytochemicals in cancer prevention: mechanism of action. J Nutr 2004;134(suppl):3479S–85S.

Lourenço R, Camilo ME. Taurine: a conditionally essential amino acid in humans? An overview in health and disease. Nutr Hosp. 2002 Nov-Dec;17(6):262-70.

Lowery LM, Devia L. Dietary protein safety and resistance exercise: what do we really know? JISSN. 2009; 6:3.

Lundin KE, Alaedini A. Non-celiac gluten sensitivity. Gastrointest Endosc Clin N Am. 2012 Oct;22(4):723-34.

Ma DF, Qin LQ, Wang PY, Katoh R. Soy isoflavone intake increases bone mineral density in the spine of menopausal women: meta-analysis of randomized controlled trials. Clin Nutr 2008;27:57–64.

Mah CD, Mah KE, Kezirian EJ, Dement WC. The effects of sleep extension on the athletic performance of collegiate basketball players. Sleep. 2011 Jul 1;34(7):943-50.

Majchrzak D, Singer I, Manner M, et al. B-vitamin status and concentrations of homocysteine in Austrian omnivores, vegetarians and vegans. Ann Nutr Metab 2006;50:485–91.

Mangravite LM, Chiu S, Wojnoonski K, Rawlings RS, Bergeron N, Krauss RM. Changes in atherogenic dyslipidemia induced by carbohydrate restriction in men are dependent on dietary protein source. J Nutr. 2011 Dec;141(12):2180-5.

Manore, M.M., M. Mason, and I. Skoog. Applying the concepts of glycemic index and glycemic loads to active individuals. ACSM Health Fitness J. 8(5):21–23. 2004.

Martarelli D, Pompei P. Oxidative stress and antioxidant changes during a 24-hours mountain bike endurance exercise in master athletes. J. Sports. Med. Phys. Fitness. 2009; 49(1):122Y7.

Martin BJ, Gaddis GM. Exercise after sleep deprivation. Med Sci Sports Exerc. 1981;13(4):220-3.

Martin BJ. Effect of sleep deprivation on tolerance of prolonged exercise. Eur J Appl Physiol Occup Physiol. 1981;47(4):345-54.

McClung JP, Karl JP, Cable SJ, et al. Randomized, double-blind, placebo controlled trial of iron supplementation in female soldiers during military training: effects on iron status, physical performance, and mood. Am. J. Clin Nutr. 2009; 90:124Y31.

McNulty H, Pentieva K, Hoey L, Ward M. Homocysteine, B-vitamins and CVD. Proc Nutr Soc 2008;67:232–7.

Meeker, D. R. & Kesten, H. D. Effect of high protein diets on experimental atherosclerosis of rabbits. Arch. Pathology 31, 147-162 (1941).

Meeker, D. R. & Kesten, H. D. Experimental atherosclerosis and high protein diets. Proc. Soc. Exp. Biol. Med. 45, 543-545 (1940).

Mellen PB, Walsh TF, Herrington DM. Whole grain intake and cardiovascular disease: a meta-analysis. Nutr Metab Cardiovasc Dis 2008;18:283–90.

Mercola J. Why Did the Russians Ban an Appliance Found in 90% of American Homes? May 2010.
http://articles.mercola.com/sites/articles/archive/2010/05/18/microwave-hazards.aspx

Messina V, Melina V, Mangels AR. A new food guide for North American vegetarians. J Am Diet Assoc 2003;103:771–5.

Miller M, Beach V, Sorkin JD, Mangano C, Dobmeier C, Novacic D, Rhyne J, Vogel RA. Comparative effects of three popular diets on lipids, endothelial function, and C-reactive protein during weight maintenance. J Am Diet Assoc. 2009 Apr;109(4):713-7.

Millward DJ. Protein and amino acid requirements of athletes. Journal of Sports Sciences, 2004, 22:143–145.

Millward DJ et al. Physical activity, protein metabolism and protein requirements. Proceedings of the Nutrition Society, 1994, 53:223–240

Molaparast-Saless F, Nellis SH, Liedkte AJ. The effects of propionylcarnitine taurine on cardiac performance in aerobic and ischemic myocardium. J Mol Cell Cardiol. 1988 Jan;20(1):63-74.

Morrison LM. Reduction of mortality rate in coronary atherosclerosis by a low cholesterol-low fat diet. Am Heart J. 1951 Oct;42(4):538-45.

Mozafar A. Enrichment of some B-vitamin in plants with application of organic fertilizers. Plant and Soil 1994;167:305-11.

Mozafar A. Is there vitamin B12 in plants or not? A plant nutritionist's view. Vegetarian Nutrition: An International Journal 1997;1/2:50-52.

Munsters, M., et al. Effects of Meal Frequency on Metabolic Profiles and Substrate Partitioning in Lean Healthy Males, PLoS One. 2012. 7(6), e38632.

Negro M, Giardina S, Marzani B, Marzatico F. Branched-chain amino acid supplementation does not enhance athletic performance but affects muscle recovery and the immune system. J. Sports. Med. Phys. Fitness. 2008; 48(3):347Y51.

Nemoseck T, Kern M. The effects of high-impact and resistance exercise on urinary calcium excretion. Int. J. Sport. Nutr. Exerc. Metab. 2009; 19(2):162Y71.

New SA. Do vegetarians have a normal bone mass? Osteoporos Int 2004;15:679–88.

New SA. Intake of fruit and vegetables: implications for bone health. Proc Nutr Soc 2003;62:889–99.

New SA et al. Dietary influences on bone mass and bone metabolism: further evidence of a positive link between fruit and vegetable consumption and bone health? American Journal of Clinical Nutrition, 2000, 71:142–151.

New SA, Millward DJ. Calcium, protein, and fruit and vegetables as dietary determinants of bone health. American Journal of Clinical Nutrition, 2003, 77:1337–1341.

Newby PK. Plant foods and plant-based diets: protective against childhood obesity? Am J Clin Nutr 2009;89(suppl):1572S–87S.

Nieman DC. Physical fitness and vegetarian diets: is there a relation? Am. J. Clin. Nutr. 1999; 70(Suppl.):570SY5S.

Nieman DC. Vegetarian dietary practices and endurance performance. Am. J. Clin. Nutr. 1988; 48:754Y61.

Nijeboer P, Mulder C, Bouma G. Non-coeliac gluten sensitivity: hype, or new epidemic?. Ned Tijdschr Geneeskd. 2013;157(21):A6168.

Norris J. Vitamin B12: Are you getting it?
http://veganhealth.org/articles/vitaminb12

Ornish D, Brown SE, Scherwitz LW, Billings JH, Armstrong WT, Ports TA, McLanahan SM, Kirkeeide RL, Brand RJ, Gould KL. Can lifestyle changes reverse coronary heart disease? The Lifestyle Heart Trial. Lancet. 1990 Jul 21;336(8708):129-33.

Ostojic SM, Ahmetovic Z. Weekly training volume and hematological status in female top-level athletes of different sports. J. Sports. Med. Phys. Fitness. 2008; 48(3):398Y403.

Pan, A. et al. Red meat consumption and mortality: results from 2 prospective cohort studies. Am. J. Clin. Nutr. 98, 1032-1041 (2013).

Phillips SM. Protein requirements and supplementation in strength sports. Nutrition. 2004; 20(7Y8):689Y95.

Pierno S, De Luca A, Camerino C, Huxtable RJ, Camerino DC. Chronic administration of taurine to aged rats improves the electrical and contractile properties of skeletal muscle fibers. J Pharmacol Exp Ther. 1998 Sep;286(3):1183-90.

Pietzak M. Celiac disease, wheat allergy, and gluten sensitivity: when gluten free is not a fad. JPEN J Parenter Enteral Nutr. 2012 Jan;36(1 Suppl):68S-75S.

Position of the American Dietetic Association and Dietitians of Canada. Vegetarian diets. J Am Diet Assoc 2003;103:748–65.

Powers SK, Jackson MJ. Exercise-induces oxidative stress: cellular mechanisms and impact on muscle force production. Physiol. Rev. 2008; 88:1243Y76.

Qin LQ, Xu JY, Wang PY, Tong J, Hoshi K. Milk consumption is a risk factor for prostate cancer in Western countries: evidence from cohort studies. Asia Pac J Clin Nutr 2007;16:467–76.

Quan R (et al). Effects of microwave radiation on anti-infective factors in human milk. Pediatrics 89(4 part I):667-669

Rahman MM, Park HM, Kim SJ, et al. Taurine prevents hypertension and increases exercise capacity in rats with fructose-induced hypertension. Am J Hypertens.2011 May;24(5):574-81.

Rana SK and Sanders TA. Taurine concentrations in the diet, plasma, urine and breast milk of vegans compared with omnivores. Br J Nutr.1986 Jul;56(1), 17-27.

Reilly T, Piercy M. The effect of partial sleep deprivation on weight-lifting performance. Ergonomics. 1994 Jan;37(1):107-15.

Ripps H, Shen W. Review: Taurine: A "very essential" amino acid. Mol Vis. 2012;18:2673-86. Epub Nov 12, 2012.

Rodenberg RE, Gustafson S. Iron as an ergogenic aid: ironclad evidence? Curr. Sports. Med. Rep. 2007; 6(4):258Y64.

Rodriguez NR, DiMarco NM, Langley S; American Dietetic Association; Dietitians of Canada; American College of Sports Medicine: Nutrition and Athletic Performance. Position of the American Dietetic Association, Dietitians of Canada, and the American College of Sports Medicine: Nutrition and athletic performance. J Am Diet Assoc. 2009 Mar;109(3):509-27. Erratum in: J Am Diet Assoc. 2013 Dec;113(12):1759

Rohrmann, S. et al. Meat consumption and mortality—results from the European Prospective Investigation into cancer and nutrition. Cancer Causes and Control 24, 685-693 (2013).

Rosell MS, Lloyd-Wright Z, Appleby PN, Sanders TAB, Allen NE, Key TJ. Long-chain n−3 polyunsaturated fatty acids in plasma in British meat-eating, vegetarian, and vegan men. Am J Clin Nutr 2005;82:327–34.

Rutherford, J., Spriet, L., et al. The Effect of Acute Taurine Ingestion on Endurance Performance and Metabolism in Well-Trained Cyclists. International

Journal of Sport Nutrition and Exercise Metabolism. August 2010. 20(4), 322-329.

Samaras TT, Storms LH, Elrick H. Longevity, mortality and body weight. Age. Res. Rev. 2002; 1(4):673Y91.

Silva, L., Silveira, P., et al. Taurine Supplementation Decreases Oxidative Stress in Skeletal Muscle After Eccentric Exercise. Cell Biochemistry and Function. January 2011. 29(1), 43-49.

Skein M, Duffield R, Edge J, Short MJ, Mündel T. Intermittent-sprint performance and muscle glycogen after 30 h of sleep deprivation. Med Sci Sports Exerc. 2011 Jul;43(7):1301-11.

Smith AM. Veganism and osteoporosis: a review of the current literature. Int J Nurs Pract 2006;12:302–6.

Song K and Milner J A. The influence of heating on the anticancer properties of garlic. Journal of Nutrition 2001;131(3S):1054S-57S

Stahler C. How many adults are vegetarian? Veg J 2006;25:14–5.

Stephens FB, Marimuthu K, Cheng Y, Patel N, Constantin D, Simpson EJ, Greenhaff PL. Vegetarians have a reduced skeletal muscle carnitine transport capacity. Am J Clin Nutr. 2011 Sep;94(3):938-44.

Stevens, M., and A. Lane. Mood regulating strategies used by athletes. J. Sport Sci. 18(1):58–59. 2000.

Stote, K., et al. A Controlled Trial of Reduced Meal Frequency without Caloric Restriction in Health, Normal-Weight, Middle-aged Adults. American Journal of Clinical Nutrition, 2007. 85(4), 981-988.

Tang JE, Phillips SM. Maximizing muscle protein anabolism: the role of protein quality. Curr. Opin. Clin. Nutr. Metab. Care. 2009; 12(1):66Y71.

Tarnopolsky MA, Atkinson SA, MacDougall JD, et al. Evaluation of protein requirements for trained strength athletes. J Appl Physiol. 1992; 73(5):1986Y95.

Tarnopolsky MA, MacDougall JD, Atkinson SA. Influence of protein intake and training status on nitrogen balance and lean body mass. J Appl Physiol. 1988 Jan;64(1):187-93.

Toohey ML, Harris MA, Williams D, Foster G, Schmidt WD, Melby CL. Cardiovascular disease risk factors are lower in African-American vegans compared to lacto-ovo-vegetarians. J Am Coll Nutr 1998;17:425–34.

Trepanowski, J., et al. Impact of Caloric and Dietary Restriction Regimens on Markers of Health and Longevity in Humans and Animals: A Summary of the Available Findings. Nutrition Journal. 2011. 10, 107.

Tucker KL, Hannan MT, Kiel DP. The acid-base hypothesis: diet and bone in the Framingham Osteoporosis Study. Eur J Nutr 2001;40:231–7.

University of Arizona, Department of Biochemistry and Molecular Biophysics, "Amino Acids Problem Set," The Biology Project, 25 Aug. 2003.

van den Berg H, Dagnelie PC, van Staveren WA. Vitamin B12 and seaweed. Lancet 1988;1:242-3.

van der Pols JC, Bain C, Gunnell D, Smith GD, Frobisher C, Martin RM. Childhood dairy intake and adult cancer risk: 65-y follow-up of the Boyd Orr cohort. Am J Clin Nutr 2007;86:1722–9.

Van Dongen HP, Maislin G, Mullington JM, Dinges DF. The cumulative cost of additional wakefulness: dose-response effects on neurobehavioral functions and sleep physiology from chronic sleep restriction and total sleep deprivation. Sleep. 2003 Mar 15;26(2):117-26. Erratum in: Sleep. 2004 Jun 15;27(4):600.

Venderley AM, Campbell WW. Vegetarian diets: nutritional considerations for athletes. Sports Med. 2006; 36(4):293Y305.

Volpe T. The fast food craze: wreaking havoc on our bodies and our animals. Parks, AZ: Volpe T Canyon Publishing, 2005.

Volta U, De Giorgio R. New understanding of gluten sensitivity. Nat Rev. Gastroenterol Hepatol. 2012 Feb 28;9(5):295-9.

Waldmann A, Koschizke JW, Leitzmann C, Hahn A. Dietary intakes and lifestyle factors of a vegan population in Germany: results from the German Vegan Study. Eur. J. Clin. Nutr. 2003; 57:947Y55.

Weaver CM. Choices for achieving adequate dietary calcium with a vegetarian diet. Am. J. Clin. Nutr. 1999; 70 (3 Suppl.):543SY8S.

Wilson AK, Ball MJ. Nutrient intake and iron status of Australian male vegetarians. Eur J Clin Nutr 1999;53:189–94.

Wójcik OP, Koenig KL, Zeleniuch-Jacquotte A, Costa M, Chen Y. The potential protective effects of taurine on coronary heart disease. Atherosclerosis. 2010 Jan;208(1):19-25.

Wolk BJ, Ganetsky M, Babu KM. Toxicity of energy drinks. Curr Opin Pediatr. 2012 Apr;24(2):243-51.

World Health Organization. Protein and Amino Acid Requirements in Human Nutrition (PDF), p. 126. 2002.

Yatabe, Y., Miyakawa, S., et al. Effects of Taurine Administration on Exercise. Advances in Experimental Medicines and Biology. 2009. 643, 245-255.

Zhang M, Izumi I, Kagamimori S, et al. Role of taurine supplementation to prevent exercise-induced oxidative stress in healthy young men. Amino Acids.2004 Mar;26(2):203-7.

Ziegenfus, T. Post-workout carbohydrate and protein supplementation. Strength Cond. J. 26(3):43–44. 2004.

Made in the USA
Middletown, DE
16 August 2015